Without warning,
Papa pivoted sharply
and slammed his fist into
her mouth. Stunned, she fell back.
Blood spurted from her lips.
Before she could move, he struck
her again and again, savagely. She
lay crumpled on the ground, barely
conscious.
Some time later—or perhaps only
minutes—she was aware of someone putting a wet cloth on her
face. A young Papago Indian
worker bent over her with concern.
"Your papa do this," he said. He
leaned down close to her face
and whispered, "You must kill him
or he will kill you."
For days afterward, Margarita
remembered the Indian boy's
words. *Kill him before he kills you.*
It made sense. If Papa were dead,
the family might have a chance to
be happy. How else could they
escape his oppressive, menacing
shadow?

THE SURGEON'S FAMILY

David Hernandez
with Carole Gift Page

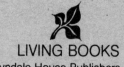

LIVING BOOKS

Tyndale House Publishers, Inc.
Wheaton, Illinois

Second printing, Living Books edition, October 1982

Library of Congress Catalog Card Number 79-66814
ISBN 0-8423-6683-0, paper
       0-8423-6684-9, Living Books Edition.

CONTENTS

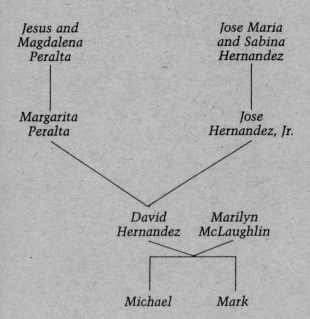

Jesus and
Magdalena
Peralta

Jose Maria
and Sabina
Hernandez

Margarita
Peralta

Jose
Hernandez, Jr.

David
Hernandez

Marilyn
McLaughlin

Michael

Mark

PROLOGUE

I, Dr. David Hernandez, have always been confident about my ability to cope, to survive. As a surgeon I have been involved with life, and death. Now I myself am dying. How will I bear this ultimate test?

Somehow I keep reflecting on my mother and father, my roots, those who bore me and made me what I am. I need to trace again the people who formed me and taught me to be a survivor.

PART ONE
THE PERALTA FAMILY

ONE
Jesus Peralta and Magdalena Duarte
Maternal Grandparents of David Hernandez

My Grandmother Magdalena was a quiet, unassuming
woman who, faithful to Mexican tradition, considered the
word of her husband law. She loved him unquestioningly in
spite of his alcoholism and fiery temper. Grandfather
Peralta was a stubborn, remote man who never really
learned how to give or receive love. I think I knew him as
well as anyone could, since he lived with my family while I
was growing up. When my mother, Margarita, learned their
full story just a few years ago, she began to understand the
tragic twists and turns her own life had taken.

When he was barely nine years old, Jesus Peralta ran away
from home. Frustration had been building within him for
many months, for nothing was as it had been. It was 1910,
the time of the Mexican Revolution. The drowsy villages of
the sprawling desert state of Sonora had been plundered,
thrown into turmoil. Imuris, the little town of Jesus' birth,
was overrun now by soldiers—rough, swaggering men who
talked bawdily, drank lustily, and swarmed like locusts over
the *barrios*, possessing the town as if it were theirs alone.

Jesus would not admit that he feared the soldiers. He
was merely . . . concerned. He and his mother lived alone,
had been alone for years—since his father, Jose Peralta, had
abandoned them and gone south to Opodepe. Time had

faded Jesus' memories of the man. Why had his father left? Because of the fighting that erupted between his parents, yes, and their constant jealousies. But why had they fought? He could not recall. He had been too young.

He knew only that now it was his place to care for his mother, to protect her. She was a lovely, vulnerable lady, and he was the man of the house. He found satisfaction in assuming such a responsibility. His mother and he managed quite well.

That is, until that disturbing night, the night the soldier came to visit. Jesus had been awakened out of sleep by noises—scuffling, his mother crying out, the soldier laughing. Jesus lay stone-still on his straw mat. Every muscle tightened as he listened intently. Was his mother in danger? Should he run to her rescue? After a minute, all was quiet except for the soldier's low, gruff voice punctuating the silence. Wait, there was more. Was Jesus mistaken, or did he hear his mother weeping?

After that night the soldier visited frequently. He was a strange, ominous man who kept his distance from the boy. Jesus hated him, although he could not say why. Finally, after many months, he understood.

His mother bore a child. A daughter.

And the soldier came to stay.

Jesus was enraged. Bitterness exploded inside him like fireworks. The taste of gall was in his mouth and fire glinted in his eyes. It was as if the Blessed Virgin had been desecrated. Surely his mother did not care for this beast of a man; she confessed as much. And yet . . . and yet! Jesus wished never to see his mother again.

So he ran to Opodepe to find his father, to begin life anew. But his father, a stranger to him now, had already remarried—a shrew of a woman nicknamed Chala. A distressed Jesus was met by the sullen, defiant stares of several young half-brothers and sisters.

Chala hated Jesus from the start. Why should this child, Jose's son by another woman, come to live in her house? She would see to it that he did not enjoy his stay. Each evening when her husband came in from the field, Chala listed her complaints.

"Can you imagine what that boy of yours has done today? Listen to his insolence! He refuses to do what I say. He must be punished!"

In anger, out of frustration, or perhaps only to appease his wife, Jose would beat his son. At times he tied the boy to a tree outside the house, flogged him mercilessly, and left him near death. Even when the blood ran freely, Jesus refused to let his father break his spirit. He held his tongue and swallowed the sobs rising in his throat. God helping him, he would take it like a man!

In spite of the persecution he received, Jesus remained in his father's house in Opodepe. Nothing could force him to go back to his mother in Imuris. Time had not dimmed his anger or his revulsion.

Over the years, in an attempt to avoid the cruelty and contempt of Chala and his half-brothers and sisters, Jesus made friends with his neighbors, Catarino and Bidala Lopez Duarte. In time, Jesus became acquainted with the entire Duarte clan. He had grown into a strikingly handsome young man with a strong, determined face, a neatly trimmed mustache, and eyes which, depending on his mood, seemed to pierce or smolder. He had learned to play the violin surprisingly well, and had become a comrade of several local musicians. He had even developed a romantic interest in Catarino Duarte's attractive daughter, Cuca.

Jesus' life might have been enjoyable now, were it not for the all-too-frequent Apache raids on the settlement. The *barrio* was distressingly vulnerable; no one knew when an Indian attack would occur. Already a number of people had been injured or killed, their possessions ravaged, and their homes destroyed. The threat of destruction and death loomed constantly.

One night Jesus awoke choking, scarcely able to breathe. Smoke filled the tiny adobe dwelling. He could hear the crackling of flames overhead, devouring the dry thatched roof. Jesus ran outside, terrified, to find the entire village being consumed in flames. He and the other villagers frantically fought the fire, but a dry desert wind carried the blaze swiftly from rooftop to rooftop.

The Duarte clan salvaged all they could from the fire, but

their spirits had taken a severe beating. The family had spent too many years warding off Apache attacks; they had lost too much, too many lives. It was time to move on.

In a voice heavy with emotion but firm in determination, Catarino told Jesus, "We can tolerate the raids no longer. We are leaving Opodepe. You have become like a son to us; you are welcome to come too."

Jesus hid his surprise. "Where—where will you go?"

"To the United States. We will go first to the border town of Nogales. When the time is right, we will cross over into Arizona."

"Who will go with you?" asked Jesus.

"Our entire family," answered Catarino. "And many who are not relatives—both workers and friends. Of course, my daughter Cuca will go . . . and her younger sister Magdalena."

Jesus carefully studied Catarino's expression. "Ah, yes, Magdalena. I have seen her often with that revolutionary Vasquez. Will he be going too?"

Catarino nodded soberly, his brow furrowed. "Yes. And—I tell you this only because you will know soon enough anyway—she carries his child."

Jesus flinched. Involuntarily he glimpsed a clear vision from the past—his mother cradling her newborn daughter, the product of that filthy scum of a soldier!

Looking away, Jesus ground his jaw harshly. Catarino's voice brought him back to the present.

"What do you say, Jesus? Will you join us?"

Jesus rubbed the bridge of his nose uncertainly. "You say Cuca is going—?"

"Yes, and many others."

"But it would mean leaving my father."

Catarino sliced the air with his hand. "Ah, your father! What has Jose Peralta ever done for you! And your half-brothers and sisters—has not the friction between you become unbearable?"

Jesus nodded reluctantly.

"Well, then," concluded Catarino, "it is settled."

"But I will go only to the border with you, and no farther," said Jesus. "I will not leave Mexico."

It was 1917 when Jesus accompanied the Duarte clan to Nogales. After a few months, in spite of his earlier resolves, he crossed over with them into Arizona. The family had no immigration papers, but since there was little monitoring at the border, papers were unnecessary.

As Jesus settled in Arizona, he felt many conflicts inside. He missed his father, regardless of what the man had done to him. There was something within Jesus that yearned for his father's respect. And now, separated from him, he would never be sure he had earned that coveted esteem. Another matter troubling Jesus just as deeply was his relationship with Cuca, which was disintegrating rapidly. He cherished her, but she had never truly loved him. As much as he hated to admit it, he was merely a diversion for her. Now she was about to marry another man. Oh, his sweet, fickle Cuca! Why had he dared to think they had a future together? Grappling with wounded vanity and inner doubts, he had an important decision to make. Should he remain in Arizona or return to his father in Opodepe?

Before Jesus could make a decision, Catarino Duarte paid him a visit. "It is over with you and Cuca, is it not?" he began.

Jesus nodded, mildly irritated. "You know that it is."

"And you have been seeing my Magdalena?"

Jesus frowned, puzzled. "We are friends. She is Cuca's sister. We talk sometimes. That is all."

Catarino thoughtfully rubbed his long, angular chin. "And what do you think of Magdalena's child?"

"What do you mean?" said Jesus. "She has a baby, a girl nearly five months old now, I suppose. Your granddaughter. What of it?"

The older man's eyes grew hard as flint. "Jesus Peralta, I want you to marry my daughter Magdalena."

Jesus drew in a breath and expelled it sharply. "Is this a joke, Catarino? She has a man, Vasquez."

"No, my son. He has gone."

"Gone? When?"

"It does not matter. What matters now is you."

Jesus turned away, angry. "Why do you ask this of me, Catarino? Why should I marry Magdalena? It is *his* baby—"

"Are you sure it is not yours, Peralta?" demanded Duarte severely.

Jesus stared in astonishment at the old man. "You know the truth, Catarino. Do not think you can involve me in your schemes!"

"My daughter has no husband," the man said levelly.

"Well, do not try to place such an obligation on me," cried Jesus. "When I look at Magdalena, I see . . . I see my—" He could not bring himself to say the word *mother*.

"This does not end the matter," said the older man bluntly. "All these years I have treated you like my own son. Very well, you cannot have Cuca, but I offer you Magdalena."

"But your Magdalena—she has no place in my heart," argued Jesus.

"No matter. Magdalena is fond of you." The man gazed cunningly at Jesus. "You know I will not rest until you take my daughter in marriage. So we will make the necessary preparations . . . unless you still refuse?"

Jesus shrugged indifferently. "I—I will not refuse you, Catarino. Why should I? I am needed nowhere else."

TWO
Margarita Peralta
Mother of David Hernandez

From her earliest childhood, my mother Margarita's afflic-
tions were exceeded only by her bravery and determination
to make something worthwhile of her life . . . and later, of
mine. Today my mother is an attractive, vivacious lady
who speaks jubilantly of her love for Christ. From her I
learned the meaning of courage.

Margarita Peralta was a large child with a wide, guileless
face, snapping dark eyes, and glowing, light brown skin. She
was naturally spirited, although she did not often smile and
she had learned early not to make demands. Her mother was
the lovely, delicate Magdalena, daughter of Catarino Duarte.
Already Magdalena's eyes were growing guardedly taciturn,
and her expression sagged in wounded resignation. She
hardly murmured a protest when her husband, Jesus Peralta,
drunk on mescal liquor or tequila, beat and berated her
child.

Margarita's earliest memories of Jesus Peralta were of a
gruff, surly man drinking heavily and spewing out a steady
stream of curses. The slightest deed could set him off, even
Margarita's innocent love pats or her artless bids for attention. "Papa, come here! Play with me, Papa!"

Inevitably he pushed her aside, his eyes glazed and voice

slurred. "Go away. I am not your papa," he would snarl. "You are not my child!"

Before Margarita learned to be wary, she embraced her father and offered kisses. "I love you, Papa," she would announce in her baffled, childish voice.

Jesus would swallow another mouthful of tequila or *pulque*, wipe his mouth with the back of his hand, and growl, "*Madre de Dios*, give me peace! I do not love this child! Tell her, Magdalena, tell her what I think of when I look at her. Tell her the truth. I am not her papa!"

When a sobbing Margarita ran imploringly to her mother, Magdalena would turn back to her weaving or to the corn tortillas she was molding. "Of course he is your papa, child," she would insist, scoffing. "Tequila fire makes him talk crazy, makes him tell big lies. Pay no attention, Margarita."

But neither mother nor daughter could long ignore the vicious, erratic behavior of Jesus Peralta. Finally it became necessary for Catarino and Bidala Duarte to take their little granddaughter into their home for protection. While there, Margarita developed a strong attachment to the family cow. Evidently the feeling was mutual, for the animal allowed the child to crawl beneath her and feed herself. Each morning the cow meandered over to the corral fence and waited patiently, motionless, while Margarita helped herself to fresh milk for breakfast.

Eventually Margarita returned to her own home. Her parents had moved from Nogales to Rillito, a railroad camp thirty miles northwest of Tucson, where Jesus worked on the Arizona lines. Magdalena, who had given birth to a second daughter, Dolores or Lola, hoped that this child might help to mellow her husband's fiery temperament. For a time the Peralta family managed to maintain a semblance of tranquillity.

One afternoon Jesus came home from the railroad and announced excitedly, "We are moving to Cortaro. They are recruiting men to lay piping for irrigation systems. New land is being opened for cotton fields. The pay will be good."

Magdalena listened quietly while her husband spoke. Then she turned from the kettle of *frijoles* she was stirring and wiped her hands on her billowing skirt. "Very well, Jesus. We will pack today."

During their first week in Cortaro, the Peraltas worked day and night to build themselves a home. Magdalena, expecting her third child, moved slowly, cumbrously, helping Jesus cut sticks from the saguaro cactus. They tied the sticks together with wire to form a square frame, then plastered the structure with mud inside and out. After the walls had dried, they made a rainproof roof of ocotillo sticks packed solidly with mud. It was an exhausting process, but worth the effort to have a home of their own.

Soon Joe Peralta was born, and later another son, Vincent. While in Cortaro, Margarita, now eight, began kindergarten—no easy task, considering the school was four miles away over a wide expanse of thickly growing mesquite. But the most harrowing aspect of this daily trek was crossing the railroad tracks on a steep twenty-foot mound. Margarita, somewhat overweight and usually lagging behind, would crawl breathlessly up the embankment, where malicious neighborhood boys often threatened to push her into the path of the oncoming train.

"Watch out, Margarita. Here comes the train!" they would tease, slapping their thighs in laughter.

"Don't fall onto the tracks, Margarita!"

"Don't roll back down the hill, Margarita!"

The train always whistled by at full, breakneck speed, the powerful rush of wind from the passing locomotive often sending the youngsters tumbling back down the hill. Margarita might have given up all hopes of crossing the tracks and attending school were it not for a friend named Rita who repeatedly helped her chase away the taunting bullies.

In 1925, Margarita no longer had to worry about crossing the ominous tracks, for the Peralta family moved away to a sprawling ranch belonging to Japanese rancher Esau Yamamoto. However, more distressing problems were about to surface.

"I am fortunate to get this job," Jesus told Magdalena as they moved their possessions into the one-room shed they would be sharing with animals, equipment, and the ranch's supply of hay. "I will handle the tractors," he continued, "and plow, and manage the irrigation systems. And did you notice the lettuce crop, Magdalena? It is magnificent. We have come upon a fine situation here."

Magdalena looked around doubtfully. Where would all the children sleep? How would anyone have even a moment of privacy? Where would she cook the meals? Another child was stirring in her belly, and she couldn't help wondering where they would put this one.

One evening after Jesus had completed his duties for Sr. Yamamoto, he came home with several companions who were clearly not regular ranch hands. Margarita and her mother exchanged wary glances. Both mother and daughter shrugged and went about their business of spreading the straw sleeping mats on the floor for the younger children. Jesus threw them a quick, cryptic glance, then spoke confidentially to his consorts.

"Liquor is very difficult to obtain these days," he said offhandedly.

"Yes, very difficult," they agreed.

"But you know where to get it," said Jesus.

"Perhaps . . . through the underground," one man said in a bland, noncommittal voice.

Jesus nodded vigorously. "Yes, that is it. You see, in Cortaro I made a great deal of liquor . . . from maize and mescal. Cactus was plentiful. We had only to gather it and dig enormous holes—"

"You made your own?" said a bearded man skeptically.

"Yes, of course."

"It was tedious work, was it not?" questioned another man, pretending indifference.

"No," said Jesus. He seemed determined to prove he was an old hand at brewing liquor. "We simply reinforced the holes with stones, heated the stones with wood—mesquite or green wood to produce the necessary temperature—and then lowered metal drums with the ingredients."

"How did you avoid discovery?"

Jesus smiled slyly. "We covered the tops with mesquite and dirt. After a few days we returned, and the mescal was ready to be fermented."

"Did you add *panocha*, brown sugar, for flavor?" quizzed the first man, catching Jesus' enthusiasm.

"Yes. And we transferred the mescal to copper bins for fifteen, maybe twenty days. Ah, the ripeness of those juices as they overflowed!"

"You had an efficient operation," observed one companion shrewdly.

"Yes, excellent," Jesus replied, his voice edged with pride.

"But not as efficient as ours," the bearded man interjected. "Don't worry, Peralta. You shall have your liquor. As much as you wish . . . for a price."

Several weeks later, while Jesus caroused with his new companions, Magdalena gave birth to another son, Ramon, a lusty, bawling, round-faced cherub. Ramon was the delight of his sister Margarita, who cared for him while her mother worked in the field. The family saw less now of Jesus, who had turned to gambling to bring in the money he needed for liquor. There were rumors, too, that Jesus was involved with other women. Some nights he came home very late; other nights he did not come home at all. But Magdalena did not question her husband. If Jesus were out somewhere drinking with his friends, or gambling, or even enjoying the favors of other women, at least he was not at home beating his wife and children. It was reason enough to say *gracias a Dios*.

In 1928, when Ramon was two years old, Margarita awoke one morning burning with fever. Her mother took one look at her and exclaimed, "Child, look at your face! You have the measles!"

The illness spread quickly through the rest of the household. One by one, Lola, the other youngsters, and finally Ramon contracted the rash. Magdalena roasted some flour and spread it on her children's skin so that they would not scratch themselves uncontrollably. In spite of her own weakness, Margarita helped constantly with her brothers and sisters, washing, feeding, and comforting them. One afternoon, while the children dozed, Magdalena gave her daughter a handful of coins and said, "We need more food and medicine. Are you too ill to walk a mile to the store?"

"I don't mind going," replied Margarita, wiping perspiration from her forehead with her sleeve. "Only the blessed saints know when Papa will come home again."

Magdalena grimaced. "Please, do not speak of your papa that way."

"But, Mama, even when he is here, he is crazy with liquor. He knows nothing anymore. What good is he?"

"Hold your tongue . . . and, *por favor*, go to the store at once. Ramon's fever burns high."

The next morning Margarita was awakened suddenly by her mother's frightened voice. "It is Ramon. He is worse. The medicine does not help."

Margarita got up quickly and gathered her feverish brother into her arms. His face was red and blotchy, his eyes glazed, unfocused. "Mama, his breathing—why is it so labored?"

Her mother twisted her hands in anguish. "It must be more than the measles. I have sent for my parents. They will know what to do."

"He will be all right, won't he?"

"I . . . I pray to the Holy Mother that he will be."

"He must be!" cried Margarita, hugging Ramon's warm, limp body against her. For hours she held him, rocked him, kissed the top of his head, cooed singsong prayers and words of endearment into his ear.

Finally her mother said, "Here, let me hold him for a while. You rest."

Margarita clutched the child possessively. "No, I will hold him."

By late afternoon Catarino and Bidala Duarte arrived. They embraced their daughter and gazed soberly at tiny, helpless Ramon.

"It is not good," said Catarino. "Where is your husband?"

"I do not know," said Magdalena.

"He is where he always is," snapped Margarita. "Drinking with his friends."

"What about Sr. Yamamoto? Surely he knows a doctor, someone who can help."

Magdalena blew cynically through her teeth. "That man? He does not care how we live or if we are well. He is fat and wealthy. He knows nothing about our needs!"

Bidala reached for Ramon. "I will take him for you, child," she told her granddaughter. "You must be weary."

Margarita drew back defensively. "No, I will not let him go."

"She has been like that all day," sighed Magdalena, brushing tears of exhaustion from her eyes.

Bidala went over to the stove and put on the iron kettle. "I will make Ramon some herb tea. It will help fight the fever. It is what my mother always used."

Margarita watched her grandmother work—a tiny, bustling woman with precise, feminine gestures. "Almost ready," said the older woman. Margarita gazed down at Ramon.

"Look, Mama," she said in surprise. "Ramon's skin is clearing. The redness is going away."

They stared at the child.

"He is not breathing," said Catarino softly.

Moments later Catarino went out in search of his son-in-law, Jesus Peralta. He knew only that Jesus was at some motel with his friends. He checked several before finally locating him, smelling of whiskey and cheap perfume. When the two men returned to the little house, Margarita, dazed and silent, still held Ramon in her arms. Magdalena sat beside them, weeping, crossing herself over and over, entreating her patron saint, *Santo Nino de Atocha*.

Jesus, unsteady, gripping Catarino's arm for support, said thickly, "Wait here. I will take care of things."

He stumbled outside and picked up a packing crate. Breaking it open with his hands, he tossed the heads of lettuce aside. Catarino squatted down to help, but Jesus waved him away. "I will do this," he said. Jesus opened another crate and discarded its lettuce, then hammered the crates together. At last he returned to the house and gently removed the child from Margarita's arms.

"Here, Ramon, my son. I have you now," he murmured. Awkwardly, tenderly, he placed the child in the narrow wooden box.

"Where will you bury him?" inquired Catarino.

"Somewhere."

"We will come too," offered Bidala.

"No, stay here. I will take care of this. He is my son."

Jesus picked up the makeshift casket and left, alone. They watched him until he was merely a shadow against the blazing Arizona sunset. No one in the family was ever to learn where the child Ramon Peralta was buried.

THREE

One day nearly a year after Ramon's death, Margarita heard a frightening commotion outside. She opened the door in time to see her father, drunk and irrational, running through the field chasing the Japanese rancher with a knife. The rancher escaped, but that evening he appeared with the authorities, who placed Jesus under arrest.

Shortly after Jesus was taken away, Magdalena slipped her shawl around her shoulders and prepared to leave. "Watch the children," she told Margarita.

"Why? Where are you going? Are you running after Papa?"

Magdalena avoided her daughter's accusing gaze. "I have business to attend to," she said crisply.

"You're going to try to get Papa out of jail! Why? He had a terrible brawl. He might have killed Sr. Yamamoto."

"I will be back," her mother replied calmly and left.

Hours later she returned to the ranch with her husband. But Sr. Yamamoto stopped Jesus before he could enter the house. "Get out, Peralta!" shouted the incensed rancher. "Pack up your family and get off my land!"

The next day the dispirited Peralta family began their journey to another ranch, this one near Glendale, Arizona. There they moved into a two-room house, spacious compared to the shed they had left behind. Magdalena was thankful for the extra room, for she was about to deliver another child. Days later she went into labor and gave birth to twins. They were stillborn. Grimly, Jesus placed the infants in two cardboard boxes and went out and buried them. Again, no one would ever know the whereabouts of the grave site. No one bothered to register the babies' births or deaths; they were simply born . . . and buried.

In 1930, Jesus Peralta was fired again, for persistent drunkenness. The family moved to still another ranch, near Benson, Arizona, where Magdalena delivered a son she named Ralph. It was a difficult delivery, but two Anglo ranchers who lived nearby summoned a doctor who was able to save the child. Jesus Peralta did not bother to come home for the birth.

Once more, he was fired from his job. This time he took his family to Sybol, a primitive railroad settlement on the east side of Tucson. At each ranch Margarita, determined to secure an education, walked three or four miles over rough terrain to attend classes. At the railroad settlement she studied in a two-room schoolhouse where the first six grades were taught together.

Often, to break the tedium of work and studies, Margarita fantasized about finding buried treasure. Rumor had it that the Indians buried jewelry and other valuables with their dead. What if she found even a few expensive ornaments or trinkets? Her family would be rich! They could escape their dreary, toilsome existence!

One night around two A.M., with visions of riches spinning in their heads, Margarita and her brother Joe sneaked out of the house and stole to a nearby Indian burial site. They dug for hours, first at one mound, then another. Unhappily, they uncovered no loot, only bones. Night after night they crept back stealthily to the graveyard in search of buried treasure. Each night they returned home disillusioned, aching with exhaustion. They reached the dismal conclusion that apparently there was no quick and easy way to get rich. Only later would Margarita realize she had gained something from the bizarre experience: she had learned not to be afraid, and she and her brother Joe had developed a special closeness she would always treasure.

In the next few years the Peralta family moved twice more, settling finally, in 1934, in Asimont, another railroad settlement, about thirty miles from Tucson. Margarita had graduated from the Benson Elementary School and was ready now for high school, but Asimont had none. Still, Margarita was determined to continue her studies. But how? Obviously her father would be no help. He was rarely sober and had no interest in the educational needs of his children.

Margarita thought about her problem each day while she cared for the younger children, and each evening when she went to Rosary with her mother. She thought about it on Saturday night when she attended the weekly railroad settlement dance. Margarita, self-taught, played the guitar, her father played his violin, and others joined them on the accordion. But even amid the frivolity, she wondered how she would complete her studies.

Then one morning she had an idea. She went to the foreman of the railroad station and told him her plight. He rubbed his chin contemplatively and replied, "My wife will pay you ten cents for six hours of work. You can wash and iron all our clothes and the children's. Mind you, we don't have any electric appliances. You'll have to do the wash by hand. And you'll have to fetch the wood yourself to heat up the stove for the iron."

"I will do it," said Margarita, smiling gratefully. "*Mil gracias*, señor!"

After completing her first day of work, Margarita returned home, exhausted but happy. But her mirth was short-lived. Her father came in drunk and irritable.

"Where have you been all day?" he demanded.

"I work now for the railroad foreman's wife."

"Who gave you permission?"

"Mama."

"What do they pay you?"

She held out her palm with the dime. He snatched it away.

"Papa, that is for my education!"

He glared at her. "You owe me a thousand times this amount for keeping you in my house!"

"No, Papa, please!"

He staggered outside. She followed, clutching at his hand. Without warning, he pivoted sharply and slammed his fist into her mouth. Stunned, she fell back. Blood spurted from her lips. Before she could move, he struck her again and again, savagely. She lay crumpled on the ground, barely conscious.

Some time later—or perhaps only minutes—she was aware of someone putting a wet cloth on her face. A young Papago Indian worker bent over her with concern. "Your mama—she is in the field. I get her," he said.

Margarita tried to speak, but her lips were too swollen.

"Your papa do this," continued the Papago youth. He leaned down close to her face and whispered, "You must kill him or he will kill you."

For days afterward, Margarita remembered the Indian boy's words. *Kill him before he kills you.* It made sense. If Papa were dead, the family might have a chance to be happy. How else could they escape his oppressive, menacing shadow?

During Margarita's next visit to the railroad station, she spied one of the foreman's guns on the counter. No one was around, so impulsively she picked it up and hid it in her shawl.

Now that she had her weapon, her plan could begin to take shape. It was just a question of the right moment. That evening, as she slipped the gun under her sleeping mat, her mother eyed her suspiciously.

"What do you have there?"

"Nothing."

"Yes, something. What is it?"

"Very well," said Margarita. "A gun."

Magdalena's face contorted slightly. "Whose gun? What will you do with a gun?"

"Never mind. It is for protection."

"From whom? Your father?"

"Yes, my father," cried Margarita, anger rising inside her. "I hate him. I want to kill him!"

Magdalena's hands flew to her mouth. She crossed herself quickly. "*Ay de mí!* You cannot do such a thing! He is my husband. I love him."

"How can you love him?" challenged Margarita. "Look how he beats you, and how we children are beaten! Still, you protect him. You support his habits. You save money for his liquor and women!" Margarita paused to catch her breath. She was trembling. She aimed her gaze squarely at her mother. "Perhaps you can tolerate him, but I cannot. I will kill him before he kills us!"

Magdalena's eyes blazed as she retorted, "The curse will be upon you forever if you do such a thing!"

Margarita was silent. It was no use discussing Papa with her mother. The matter was closed. Margarita would do what she had to do.

A few days later, as Margarita started home after finishing her chores for the foreman's wife, she noticed a strange flurry of activity near the Asimont station. She heard guitar music and singing. A number of Papago Indians had clustered a short distance from a group of musicians. Papago women and children stood cautiously in the doorways of their huts or stared curiously out their windows.

Margarita approached the musicians, fascinated. Their music was different from anything she had heard before. As she listened, one man stepped forward and smiled. "Do you like our song?" he asked.

"What is it?"

"It is called *Nitido Rayo por Cristo*. Let me teach it to you."

Margarita shrugged, a bit embarrassed. "I like the sound, but what is it all about?"

"It is about Jesus," said the man. "Do you believe in Jesus?"

Margarita nodded solemnly. "I do believe. My mother has many saints in our house. I have Jesus, Mary, Joseph, the apostles, and other patron saints."

The man shook his head vigorously. "No. I am talking about Jesus Christ, the Son of God. No man comes to the Father except through his Son."

Margarita gazed without comprehension at the stranger, then turned her attention back to the compelling music.

Later, as the group prepared to leave, the man approached Margarita again. "I am Brother Morales from the Mexican

Baptist Church in Tucson," he said. "I would like to give you this hymnbook and a Bible. We will return next month. Please come see us again."

Margarita accepted the books with silent astonishment. She went home and began to read her new Bible, but she found the words difficult to understand. Still, she resolved to keep reading. One day her mother discovered the Bible and grabbed it away, furious.

"Where did you get this?" she demanded.

"From Brother Morales," replied Margarita.

Viciously her mother tore the Bible apart. "Those people are diabolical," she cried. "They are 'hallelujahs.' I want you to stay away from them!"

Margarita was silent. She would promise no such thing. The next month, when Brother Morales and his team returned to Asimont, Margarita asked them for a second Bible.

This one, too, her mother destroyed.

For the third time Brother Morales gave Margarita a Bible. During this visit, he talked to her about God's love.

Love? What is love? wondered Margarita. *God's love? What a strange concept.* She had never seen God's love in her home, nor among the people who lived in the settlements.

"Jesus loves you," Brother Morales told her earnestly.

Margarita began to cry. How could Jesus love her? She was full of hatred for her father; she even planned to kill him. Surely God could not love her.

But Brother Morales insisted that God did, and that Margarita could know him personally. Was it possible that here was her opportunity to escape the tragedy and chaos that surrounded her? Surely something better existed beyond the despair, the poverty, the drunkenness and superstition that engulfed her life.

"I would like to know this Jesus you speak of," she told Brother Morales.

That afternoon Margarita studied her Bible with fresh enthusiasm, wanting to learn all she could about her new Savior. Opening the book at random, she read a verse: "Vengeance is mine, saith the Lord."

The idea was new, challenging, totally against everything Margarita had ever heard or witnessed or experienced. But God said it, so she would obey. She would do nothing to harm her father. The next day she returned the gun to the Asimont station.

Margarita hid her Bible from her mother and studied it alone behind the desert brush, often stealing out after midnight with a flashlight, to read. But an unexpected situation was developing—an estrangement between mother and daughter. Margarita felt bewildered. She and her mother had always been so close, but now Mama seemed to have turned on her. The rift between them intensified when Margarita refused to attend Rosary with Magdalena. The angry woman gripped her daughter's arm and slapped her repeatedly, shouting, "This will get the devil out of you!"

The next time Brother Morales visited Asimont, Margarita told him of her desire to attend high school. "I see the futility and agony of my parents' way of life," she explained. "The station foreman has arranged for me to receive a twenty-five cent allotment each week from the National Relief Act to attend school in Tucson. But I have no place to stay."

Brother Morales and his wife exchanged smiles and nodded. "You are welcome to stay in our home in Tucson and attend school," he said, "at least until you are able to make other arrangements."

But later, when Margarita broached the subject with her mother, Magdalena growled her contempt. "I do not understand why you wish to abandon us to go to school. We need you here. *I* need you."

"I will come back next summer, Mama, when I have completed ninth grade," she replied, forcing a lightness into her voice.

Margarita spent three months in the Morales home, then moved in with Sister Villegas, an elderly deaconess for whom she cooked and cleaned. Margarita worked diligently, combining studies with long, arduous hours of housework. But the woman remained critical and unappreciative, daily inspecting every nook and cranny of her house for dust. The eccentric lady spent most of her time in her rocking chair reading the Bible and smoking cigarettes. Her Bible was scarred with burns and ashes, but she clung stubbornly to her tobacco.

Brother Morales had secured this position for Margarita, but he never returned to see how she fared. Margarita's spirits sagged. She felt confused. She had not expected to see imperfect Christians, selfish and undisciplined, often lacking love and concern. And the financial burden was mounting, for her father took and squandered her monthly allotment from the NRA before she could receive it from the station foreman.

When summer arrived, Margarita returned to her family in Asimont. As she had anticipated, she felt as if she were stepping back into the clutches of a nightmare. She made the best of the situation, carting the children to church in Tucson each Sunday in the family's old Model-T. Each Saturday she washed, ironed, and mended the youngsters' clothing in preparation for Sunday school.

One Saturday night in May would etch itself in her memory forever. Late in the evening she ironed the last of the children's clothing. It had been a long day—heating water in the old wash tub, scrubbing and starching the clothes, then heating the iron on the wood-burning stove. Margarita wiped her brow and wondered if she would collapse before the work was done.

Suddenly she heard a disturbance outside the door. Jesus Peralta burst inside with his drinking companions, shouting and cursing. Her mother stood to quiet him, gesturing toward the sleeping area. "The children, Jesus. They are sleeping."

Incoherent, nearly delirious, Jesus threw Magdalena to the floor and began to beat her violently. In desperation Margarita jumped on his back and pounded him with her fists. "Leave my mother alone!" she screamed.

Enraged, Jesus lurched backward, upsetting Margarita. She lay dazed, sprawled on the floor beside her mother, who whimpered softly now. Jesus sent his comrades outside, then placed a metal bar on the door. Pulling a leather rope from the waist of his trousers, he turned and lumbered toward Margarita, his expression rabid. He raised the strap and snapped it viciously across her back, then again. Ugly red stripes appeared on her white cotton blouse. Margarita scrambled out of his reach, but he pursued her doggedly. As she crawled toward the stove, he kicked her in the stomach. Recoiling in pain, she pulled herself into the corner, behind the little aluminum stove.

It dawned on her that he had her cornered now. This was it. He would kill her for sure.

"Magdalena," he bellowed, "fire up the stove with those railroad ties!" When she hesitated, he glared at the ax leaning against one wall. Magdalena saw it too and shuddered. Without a word, she obeyed and brought the kindling.

As the fire blazed, the sides of the stove reddened and oil from the railroad ties filled the room with black, foulsmelling smoke. Margarita, struggling for breath, pressed her body against the wall in a futile attempt to avoid the scorching heat.

"More wood!" shrieked her father. He picked up a gallon jug of whiskey and guzzled lustily. "Stoke it again!" he demanded, wiping the liquor from his mouth with his shirt sleeve.

The heat was nearly unbearable now. Blisters erupted on Margarita's arms and legs. "O God, save me!" she cried aloud. "Don't let him harm me. Save me from this hell!"

Her father laughed cynically. "Go on. Call out to that God of yours. See if he can save you!" He threw a glance at his cowering wife and ordered her to stoke the fire again. Once more he lifted the jug and drank greedily. He squinted at Margarita and said tauntingly, "Where is this God you call after? Do you think he can help you?"

Margarita sobbed, choking convulsively on the dense, suffocating fumes. The heat was searing her flesh. The pain was excruciating. Her knees were about to buckle.

She caught a glimpse of her father raising his bottle exultantly. Suddenly the jug slipped from his fingers and crashed on the floor, shattering noisily. In disbelief he stared down at the pool of liquid. "That's all there was," he blurted thickly. Cursing and blaspheming, he stumbled to the door, threw down the bar, and stomped out of the house. A minute later, they heard him roar off into the night in his Model-T.

FOUR

In a frenzy, Magdalena threw water on the blazing stove, while Margarita darted out of the hot, blackening corner. Trembling with relief, she splashed water on her face and arms, then turned sharply to confront her mother. "You know Papa is going to Tucson for more whiskey."

Magdalena nodded, her expression grave.

"When he returns, I will be gone," said Margarita breathlessly. "If you want to join me, come along. If not, stay. But I'm leaving."

Somberly Magdalena rubbed a massive bruise on her upper arm. "I—I will go with you," she said at last, lowering her head in mournful resignation.

Margarita sprang into action. She roused five-year-old Ralph and eight-year-old Vincent. Joe and Lola, who had awakened and overheard the conversation, were already gathering their few possessions.

"Where will we go?" asked Lola excitedly.

"To Tucson," replied Margarita.

"But Papa took the car," said Joe.

"So we will walk."

"It is thirty miles."

"No matter."

"It is the middle of the night."

Margarita remained firm. "We must get out before Papa returns."

Magdalena held out a few scraps of two-day-old tortillas. "This is all the food we have to take with us."

Nudging the children out the door, Margarita replied, "Bring them, Mama. They are better than nothing."

For hours the impromptu troupe wended their way through desert mesquite and over broken terrain, avoiding the road lest they encounter a drunken, violent Jesus Peralta. Surely he would kill them all for daring to flee.

Around four A.M. they approached a dry irrigation canal and followed it to a ranch. The area was parched, the children thirsty. Margarita ran a mile ahead in search of water. By the time she returned, the morning sun was a red arc on the horizon.

"The children are cold," Magdalena told her plaintively.

Margarita knelt down and scooped up some sand. "Look, Mama. It is still warm with yesterday's sun. We could cover them with it like a blanket."

The children took quickly to the idea, burrowing down like moles into the loose, shifting granules. Shortly one could see only smiling faces peering from great mounds of sand.

Margarita gazed toward the ranch on a craggy bluff above them. An idea was brewing. She turned to her mother. "Take off your gold earrings. I have a plan."

Magdalena touched her earlobes unconsciously. "These earrings are not real gold."

"We have no money. They will do."

Margarita scaled the rocky incline to the ranch and knocked vigorously on the thick oak door. A man answered.

"Please, señor, I need food for my mother and my brothers and sisters," said Margarita.

His eyes narrowed suspiciously. "No. I have nothing. Go away."

Margarita held out the earrings. "These are gold. I will give them to you for food."

"What you ask is illegal. I'm sorry." The door closed loudly.

Margarita walked a short distance from the house and waited. Eventually the man came out and disposed of the garbage. When he had gone back inside, Margarita crept over furtively and scavenged the leftovers. She carried them back to her family like a costly prize. They would have breakfast after all!

With renewed strength, they walked ten miles to the next railroad settlement. Here, Margarita again offered the earrings for food. A generous Mexican family agreed, bringing out *frijoles*, tortillas, and fruit for the hungry travelers.

They set out again on the highway from Benson to Tucson, hitching a ride with a sympathetic construction foreman. In Tucson, Magdalena insisted they go to the home of her cousin. The relative invited them to stay. The next day Margarita went out looking for work. A Jewish man gave her a job cleaning and sorting shoes in his shoe store for three dollars a month. But Margarita worked with such diligence that he gave her two dollars for her first week's salary.

During the family's second week in Tucson, Margarita suspected that her mother was in touch with her father. When Margarita returned from work one afternoon, her mother said, "Your father is circling the house."

Margarita eyed her mother warily. "You contacted him, didn't you? You told him where we are." When Magdalena made no reply, Margarita's temper flared. "If he comes back into our lives, I will not remain here!"

"But where will we go? We have no money and no car."

"I will find a way," resolved Margarita. She thought a moment. "They are taking truckloads of families— 'renganches'—to the cotton fields, under contract. Perhaps we—"

"No!" cried Magdalena. "I would rather go back to Asimont!"

"Back to Papa?"

"He has promised he will change, if only we give him another chance."

"How can you believe him, after all he has done to us?"

"He even says he will drive us to Tucson every Sunday for church. Please," urged her mother, "we must go home."

Tears of frustration burned in Margarita's eyes. "You will not listen to me. You see only Papa's way. I will go back, but we shall see if things are different!"

As Margarita feared, Jesus Peralta had not changed. For a few weeks he drove his family to the Baptist church (even Magdalena was attending now), but inevitably he returned for them in a drunken stupor. Finally he refused to take them to Tucson, and the beatings began again.

One morning, out of desperation, Margarita took her father's Model-T and fled with her family to Tucson. After hiding the car at the home of Magdalena's cousin, they joined the "*renganches*," traveling by truck to the cotton fields of Casa Grande. The ranch manager provided them with a tent in a desolate area of the camp where rattlesnakes abounded. Sleeping on the floor, Magdalena and the children awoke many mornings to find fresh rattlesnake markings in the soil around their bedding. Cooking utensils had to be inspected every morning, since the snakes seemed to delight in curling leisurely inside pots and pans.

A month passed. Then one evening, as Margarita and her brother Joe trudged home from the field, she said, "It's time to move on. School will be starting soon."

Joe agreed. "Mama says Papa knows where we are. He may come any time."

The next day the two hitched a ride on a truck going to Tucson, picked up the Model-T, and drove back to the cotton ranch. But for Margarita, that overnight trip back to Casa Grande was a terrifying ordeal. The road paralleled the railroad tracks where countless vagabonds and drifters camped and built small bonfires while waiting to hop a train. Margarita had heard gruesome tales of rape, assault, and robbery occurring along this barren stretch of desert. Every hobo's fire represented a threat. What if someone tried to stop her vehicle? What if the car broke down? While she fretted through the seemingly endless night, Joe slept peacefully beside her. At daybreak, they arrived safe and sound—to Margarita's immense relief—and found Mama curled against a large rock at the ranch entrance, waiting. She had been there all night.

That day they collected their earnings, packed everything

into the automobile, and headed for Phoenix where Grandmother and Grandfather Duarte lived.

A few days later, Grandfather Duarte found them a little two-room house in "Ragtown," the ghetto section of Phoenix also known as *El Barrio de las Ilachas*, or "The Dirty Sock." Margarita began attending an evangelical Baptist church pastored by Brother Leonardo Mercado. She worked six days a week as a field hand, leaving on a truck at dawn to pick cotton, carrots, or strawberries, or to pack lettuce. She returned late every evening; she had no choice if her family was to survive.

Two months after their arrival in Phoenix, Jesus Peralta found them again. Margarita faced her mother and demanded, "How did he know where we were?"

"It's none of your business," said the woman.

Margarita wouldn't be put off. "Tell me how, Mama. You can't read or write. Did you hire someone to send him a letter in Asimont? Surely that has to be it!"

"It does not matter. He is here. We must make the best of it."

Margarita relinquished her anger. What good would it do to turn against her mother? It was obvious that Magdalena's devotion to Jesus Peralta would never die.

One Saturday after an especially distressing clash with her father, Margarita stayed overnight with her Grandmother and Grandfather Duarte. Early Sunday morning she dressed for church, slipping into her nicest outfit—a lacy, ankle-length dress with ruffled sleeves. Seriously she contemplated her reflection in her grandmother's mirror. Except for the fresh bruise on her right cheek, she felt pleased with her appearance.

Sometime during the past couple of years, spent working the fields, studying diligently, and running from her father, Margarita had become a woman. Her figure was trim; she had warm, smiling eyes, full lips, and finely arched brows. Her short, velvety hair waved attractively around her oval face. Lately young men had begun seeking out her attention. She enjoyed their approving glances, their compliments. It was flattering to have admirers.

As Margarita patted a curl into place, she became aware of

an insistent pounding on the door—and her father's boozy, outraged shouts, demanding that she come outside. "You child of a slut!" he stormed. "I will teach you to ridicule me!"

Margarita heard her grandparents open the door and try in vain to quiet the crazed man. Swiftly she put on her high-heel shoes and stole out the back door. As she hurried north on 16th Street toward the church, she glanced back anxiously. Just as she feared, her father had spotted her and was in heated pursuit—and he was carrying a chain!

She broke into a run. A long shrill whistle sounded in the distance. The nine A.M. freight train was approaching the 16th Street crossing just one-half block ahead. She could see the train now—a grimy giant exploding toward her, monstrous, deafening.

Behind her, Jesus Peralta was edging perilously close. Panic seized her. She would be trapped between him and the passing train, murdered on the spot, unless somehow she beat the train. Her heart raced as she sprinted desperately toward the crossing. Her high-heels felt like lead on the rough cobblestone. Her legs ached beyond endurance.

"O God, please rescue me," she gasped breathlessly, urgently. "You know how much I wish to serve you. Allow me to reach the crossing before the train!"

There was but an instant to choose. Behind her, a brutal, hellish man flailed the air with his ominous chain. Ahead, a massive engine bore down rapidly and was almost upon her.

A chilling childhood recollection stabbed her consciousness—malicious boys threatening to push her in front of a train. Her imagination burst with the familiar nightmare—the hideous thud of impact, her body flung skyward, broken.

The terrifying vision vanished as she sprang daringly—a dizzying leap just in front of the onrushing locomotive. The air cushion lifted her skirt as the train roared past. The whistle screamed. Paroxysms of movement convulsed the earth while the huge boxcars rumbled by, a few scant feet away.

She was safe. *Thank God*! She sighed her relief and struggled to catch her breath. Pushing back her tousled hair and smoothing her skirt, she scurried on across Eastlake Park to Sunday school. She did not reveal her harrowing experience to anyone in the congregation. For now, she was content just to be in God's house, safe, alive.

But Margarita had not escaped her father's wrath for long. In the week that followed, he severely thrashed her and her mother. The next Sunday, suffering from a mild concussion, Margarita fainted in church.

Several weeks later, her parents decided to move to Glendale, Arizona. Margarita chose to remain in Phoenix, to avoid her father's abusive behavior and to stay close to her church where she served as president of the young people's group. In fact, her social life revolved around Brother Mercado's church. She attended Sunday morning and evening services, Tuesday youth get-togethers, Wednesday night prayer meetings, and weekend planning activities. Were it not for her relationship with Christ and her fellowship with God's people, Margarita likely would have succumbed to despair.

When her parents left for Glendale, Margarita accepted a position as live-in maid for a local family. Both husband and wife worked. But the job ended abruptly after only one month when Margarita faced an unexpected dilemma. One evening the wife attended a society party while her husband remained at home. Margarita was caring for the two children in her own room. Suddenly the husband entered. "I just wanted to check on the children," he said.

"They are getting sleepy," she replied.

"Time for bed then." The man drew near and lightly ran his hand over Margarita's arm. "Then perhaps you and I could spend some time together—"

Margarita forced herself to remain calm. "I have much work to do."

His fingers traveled to her neck, her hair. "You are very lovely, Margarita. So very lovely."

She eased away from his touch. "I really must get the children to bed." She picked up one drowsy toddler and laid him in his crib.

After several uneasy moments, Margarita persuaded the man to leave the room. Swiftly she dressed the youngsters for bed, then gathered her few belongings. She slipped quietly out the back door into the chill, uninviting night, grimly concluding that all men were indeed as menacing as her own father. Where to now? she wondered. There was only one answer—to her parents' new home in Glendale.

She should have known better. Her father proved to be as venomous and irrational as ever. Eventually Margarita returned to Phoenix with her mother and her brothers and sisters, and rented a tiny house close to the church. But the family's peace was short-lived. In a few months Jesus Peralta arrived and, dismayingly, picked up where he left off.

Meanwhile, Margarita's attention was turning increasingly away from her family and the insurmountable problems at home. She had begun dating Tony Soza, a handsome, intelligent young man with a good job. The perfect gentleman, he always treated her with kindness and consideration. Clearly, he adored her.

But Margarita was too skeptical to appreciate Tony's tender qualities and rashly broke up with him. Only a teenager still "spreading her wings," she had little firsthand knowledge of loyalty or committed love. She considered romance a game, not to be taken too seriously.

But if Margarita admitted the truth, she mistrusted everyone; she assumed all people had ulterior motives. Surely they were after something or out to do her harm. And the painful question surfaced again, How could she be sure all men were not, in essence, like her father?

While she was dating Tony, Margarita became acquainted with another young man, Jose Hernandez, a recent convert who had been baptized on Easter Sunday, 1936. She saw him at church and sometimes they worked together in the field. He was dating a sweet girl named Lucy. Just as well, too, for Margarita certainly wasn't attracted to him. Fastidious about her own appearance, Margarita thought Jose rather careless in his dress and not the most handsome fellow. Nevertheless, he had character traits and principles which far surpassed her first superficial impressions of him. And, too, they shared a dubious bond. Like hers, his home life was far from satisfactory.

One weekend in May, the young people went out to cut

flowers from the gardens of various church members in preparation for the Mother's Day services. Pausing in his work, Jose strode over to Margarita, his manner brisk and straightforward. "I understand you have broken up with Tony," he observed. "I myself have stopped seeing Lucy. Would you like to be my girl friend?"

"Sure," she replied. The word tumbled out automatically.

"Oh, but wait a minute," he continued. "I don't expect a thoughtless or flimsy reply."

"No?" questioned Margarita lightly. She continued to pick the flowers.

"I'm different from your other admirers," he persisted. "I'll give you fifteen days to pray and think seriously about this decision."

"Fifteen days?" she echoed with amusement. "Why, I can answer you right now."

He remained firm, his expression sober. "You may answer all the others glibly, Margarita, but not me. I will pray, too, because I want you to be my girl friend . . . but I also want you for my wife."

Margarita looked up, dumbfounded. Never had any of her previous boyfriends mentioned marriage. Surely this bold young man was speaking in jest.

But fifteen days later, true to his word, Jose Hernandez approached Margarita for her answer. She had prayed and pondered and even consulted her mother, asking, "What do you think, Mama? Should I get married?"

Magdalena had responded with anger and alarm. "No, you cannot! We need you here with us!"

But Margarita refused to be swayed by her mother's impassioned arguments. Desperate for a new life, a fresh start, she was ready to commit herself to this capable, commanding young man, Jose Hernandez.

PART TWO
THE HERNANDEZ FAMILY

FIVE

Jose Maria Hernandez
Paternal Grandfather of David Hernandez

*Like my mother, my father, Jose Hernandez, had learned to
live with a harsh, strong-willed father who considered
physical thrashings the basis of all discipline. In fact, while
my mother and father were dating, they often compared
their beatings and bruises. While my father was—and is—a
sober, reticent man of unquestionable principles, his father,
Jose Maria, was a rapscallion of sorts—a bold, feisty,
outspoken fellow whose life was marked by violence and
pride. A man of few words, he rarely showed affection, but
his ambition and cunning were irrepressible. He was first
and last, a survivor. There was a time, however, many years
ago, when it looked quite doubtful that my grandfather Jose
Maria would survive at all.*

Jose Maria Hernandez, a short, solidly built man in his
twenties, ran breathlessly along the narrow, cobbled streets
of Villa Unión, a village just south of Mazatlan. He passed
the white adobe buildings with wrought-iron balconies and
the stone walls spilling over with lush, blooming bougain-
villea and jacaranda. Reaching the marketplace, he gazed
intently at the open-air food stands and the stalls displaying
brightly colored tapestries, pottery, and wicker baskets. His
brother was nowhere in sight.

"Have you seen Marciano?" he asked a boy leading a burro laden with baskets of peyote.

"Perhaps the *cantina*?" suggested the youth.

Jose Maria glanced toward the saloon and nodded. "*Gracias, muchacho.*" He strode toward the timeworn building with its grilled windows and carved panel door. An elderly woman, her pinched, leathery face partly hidden by her shawl, held out a basket of onions, oranges, and peppers. "*Se vende frutas. Se vende legumbres,*" she said plaintively.

"*No gracias,*" señora," said Jose Maria impatiently, pushing open the door.

"*Dos centavos,* señor," she called after him in a sad, wheedling voice. He didn't look back.

Inside, Jose Maria spotted his brother sitting at a table with several companions who filled the room with braying laughter.

"Marciano!" said Jose Maria.

Marciano looked up, startled, and put down his mug of tequila. "Jose Maria!"

"I have news. Come with me."

Marciano held up his thumb and forefinger, measuring a quarter-inch of space. "*Momentito,*" he replied with a grin.

"No, now," said Jose Maria. "It is about the fiesta tonight."

"Ah, yes. Our wives have talked about nothing else for days," laughed Marciano. "Such a celebration it will be!"

"Mama Elena fears our brother Domingo will announce his engagement to Maria tonight," interjected Jose Maria.

Marciano's mouth opened in surprise. "I did not think Domingo was so serious about the girl. Besides, Maria's family will be at the festivities."

"Domingo admits he cares for Maria, and he says he is not afraid of her family."

"But her brothers hate us," argued Marciano. "I think they are jealous of our warehouses, our cattle and land."

"It is foolishness," scoffed Jose Maria. "We are not so rich."

"Still, they will never permit a marriage between our families."

"I know your brother Domingo," remarked one of Marciano's drinking companions. "He is an astronomer. He teaches in the school here. He is a very smart man, your brother."

"Yes, smart," agreed Jose Maria, sitting down at the table beside Marciano and helping himself to a jug of *pulque*. "I only hope love has not dulled Domingo's senses."

"I knew your father too," continued the man opposite Jose Maria. "Benceslau Hernandez, a fine architect. Without equal in all Sinaloa."

"Yes, a very good man, my father," nodded Marciano. "And an astute businessman. They called him 'Rey de Cuero' because of his tough hide."

The men laughed.

As one fellow poured more tequila, he observed, "I recall that some time ago your father was thrown by a mad burro and killed. How does your mother fare since his death?"

Jose Maria smiled. "Mama Elena always fares well. She is a strong woman and as clever as any man. She manages our family's brick and tile business very well."

Marciano nudged his brother. "Don't forget. She has us to supervise the masons and carpenters."

"*Qué lástima!* We are kept too busy for mischief," chuckled Jose Maria. He finished his drink and stood up. Gazing at Marciano, his expression shifted into an unmistakable frown. "Mama Elena frets herself over Domingo. Our younger brother is a man who lives by his heart and his brains, not by his fists like you and I, Chano," he said, using the affectionate tag the family had given Marciano. "Let us keep our eyes on Domingo tonight at the fiesta."

Marciano, in turn, responded with Jose Maria's family name. "Don't worry, Chema," he said, raising his drink in salute, "if need be, I will send my *mozos*, my personal servants and guards, to protect our brother."

That evening Jose Maria and Marciano, with their wives Sabina and Hortencia, accompanied Domingo to the fiesta. The plaza in the center of town was already crowded with ladies in their prettiest dresses and men wearing handsome *serapes*. The bandstand was decorated with orchids and azaleas. There were tables brimming with roasted turkeys and chickens, papayas and pineapples, bananas and mangos. The aroma of *frijoles* and fried tortillas wafted on the air.

Domingo helped himself to some papaya, then stood watching the *mariachis* in their trim black trousers and short jackets with glittering buttons. The musicians strolled among the couples, singing and strumming their guitars, several playing trumpets or violins.

When Domingo spotted Maria, he greeted her with a kiss and took her in his arms. They danced gaily, energetically, losing themselves in the rhapsodic music. Even when Maria's incensed brother Juan rudely broke in on them, Domingo remained unruffled.

But the angry young man would not be ignored. "Domingo Hernandez, leave my sister alone!" Juan demanded.

"She has something to say about that," replied Domingo.

"No. I speak for her . . . and for my family."

"You speak for no one," hissed Maria. "I speak for myself. I love Domingo."

Juan gripped Maria's arm and pulled her close until their faces nearly touched. "Did you know your Domingo has another girl friend? A young teacher in Embocada. They are having an affair."

Maria broke away and spat on the ground at Juan's feet. "This is what I think of your lies! I will never stop loving Domingo!"

Juan's brows furrowed menacingly and his nostrils flared. "You will regret those words, Maria."

Without warning, Domingo's brother Jose Maria stepped forward and eyed Juan coldly. "*Retírese de aquí, amigito!*"

"You heard him, Juan," echoed Maria. "Go home. Leave me alone!"

The youth stood his ground momentarily, glowering at the two Hernandez brothers. "It is not yet over between us," he warned, then pivoted and stalked away.

Trembling, Maria slipped into Domingo's arms and murmured, "Why—why is Juan so jealous?"

Domingo embraced her protectively. "It makes no sense, *querida*. He behaves more like your lover than your brother."

Jose Maria gripped his brother's shoulder in a gesture of comradeship and concern. "Watch out for that one, Domingo. He brings nothing but trouble."

Several days after the fiesta, Domingo left early one morning for Mazatlan, where he would receive a teaching assignment for the northern town of Culiacan. As noon approached, Mama Elena anxiously watched the road for Domingo's return. It was the rainy season, and a servant had reported that the river had inundated the road entering Villa Unión, the very route Domingo would be traveling.

"Mama Elena, I will ride across the river and take a horse for Domingo," suggested her youngest son, nine-year-old Topio.

The woman nodded. "Go, but be careful, my son."

Minutes later Topio mounted his horse and rode eagerly toward the outskirts of town. He crossed the river just as a weary Domingo shuffled toward the water's edge. The two grinned as their eyes met.

"How pleased I am to see you, Topio!"

"More pleased to see the horse, I think," teased the boy.

Domingo climbed on his mount and flicked the reins. The horses trotted surefootedly back through the muddy, flowing river.

Several blocks from the river the two brothers passed the *Cubertizo*, a saloon in the business section of Villa Unión. Suddenly a man's voice broke the stillness. "Domingo, is that you?"

Domingo pulled on his mare's reins and stared at three men emerging from the saloon. Maria's brothers!

"Domingo, come in and have a drink with us," called Juan, his voice thick and truculent. He stood stubbornly in the way of Domingo's pawing mare.

"You know I'm not a drinker," replied Domingo. "Let us pass."

"Don't be impolite, Domingo. We have waited a long time for you to arrive."

"I am on my way home. Let me by."

"Or on your way to see Maria perhaps?" taunted Juan. Another brother stepped forward and reached up to pull Domingo from his saddle.

Topio, realizing a fight was imminent, dug his heels into his horse and sprinted off toward home. He rode furiously, then sprang from the animal and burst in the door of Jose Maria's hacienda just off the main ranch house. It was siesta time, and Jose Maria was resting on his bed in his long cotton underwear while his young son, Jose Maria Jr., played contentedly on the floor beside him.

"Chema, Chema, *levantate pronto!*" cried Topio. "They are beating up Domingo!"

"Where?"

"At the *Cubertizo!*"

Jose Maria jumped off the bed, pulled on his trousers, grabbed his sawed-off machete, and dashed out the door. Topio ran to the main house to alert Mama Elena and his sisters Jovita and Victoria. Shortly he caught up with Jose Maria on the road.

"Marciano is still away on business and will not return until late this evening," Topio cried breathlessly.

By the time Jose Maria and Topio arrived at the saloon, a crowd was gathering. Spotting Maria's brothers, Jose Maria strode toward them, demanding, "Where is Domingo?"

In one swift motion Juan drew a knife and ripped open Jose Maria's abdomen. Jose Maria stared down in shock at his exposed intestines. Holding the protruding entrails with one hand, Jose Maria swung his machete. A stricken Juan, his face registering surprise, crumpled soundlessly, dead. A second brother sprang in attack. Jose Maria lurched toward him and struck blindly with his machete, slicing off the youth's right ear and severing his arm at the shoulder. Maria's third brother, called "El Guerro," ran in retreat, with young Topio close on his heels.

"No, no, Topio!" Jose Maria cried. Then, weakened by his own blood loss, he slumped on the ground, unconscious.

Moments later Mama Elena arrived with her two daughters. She rushed to Jose Maria, wailing, "Chema! My Chema!" Seeing that he was still alive, she crossed herself in relief. Then she spotted Domingo lying face down in the dirt nearby. She scurried to him, turned him over, and cradled his head in her arms. "*Hijo mio*—my son!" she wept.

Domingo's eyes fluttered open momentarily. He smiled

and his lips parted as if he might speak. Then, wordlessly, he died.

A deep, guttural moan rose from the woman. "*No te apures, hijo.* I will avenge your life with my own hand," she vowed.

While Mama Elena embraced her lifeless son, seven-year-old Victoria fell on her knees beside Jose Maria and wept helplessly. Jovita, the oldest daughter, knelt and prayed in a soft, urgent voice.

"We have called for the doctor," someone told them. "Surely he will come quickly."

Near a corner of the building, Maria's severely wounded brother twisted in agony. Seeing Victoria, he stretched out his remaining arm and called, "Please, little girl, save me, save me, for your brother will kill me!"

"He can kill no one lying here like this," retorted Victoria.

Victoria's angry voice roused Mama Elena from her paralysis of grief. She released Domingo and returned to Jose Maria. Rolling him over, she saw that his gaping wound was glutted with dirt.

"Where is the doctor!" she demanded.

"*Estoy aquí*—I am here," replied a young man wending his way through the hovering throng. He bent down, briefly examined Jose Maria, then stood up and shook his head. "*Lo siento.* There is nothing I can do. He is dying."

"You must treat him," insisted Mama Elena.

"I am only a medical student, señora, not yet fully trained. The dirt in your son's wound will kill him."

Desperately Mama Elena gripped the man's arm. "*Por favor, en el nombre de Dios!* I have lost one son today. I will not lose another!"

The man pulled away. "I cannot risk my life for a dying man. His enemies may avenge themselves on me."

Mama Elena gazed dolefully at her son. Then, on impulse, she leaned forward and struggled to stuff the bulging intestines back inside his abdomen—a nearly impossible task. Somehow she managed it. Whipping off her shawl, she wrapped it snugly around Jose Maria's middle. She looked up, perspiration beading on her face. "*Por favor,* someone bring the local authorities," she cried imploringly. "I want my son taken immediately to Mazatlan. There they will treat him."

At last the townspeople began to rally, perhaps recalling Elena Hernandez' influence and wealth. Her wishes were carried out promptly now. Both her son Jose Maria and Maria's wounded brother were transferred by train, under guard, to a hospital in Mazatlan. Mama Elena sent Jovita and Victoria with Jose Maria. "Get the best doctors," she instructed before the train pulled away, "and tell them I will pay generously. I will join you after I have found Topio and warned Marciano."

Several men in the crowd carried Domingo's body back to the ranch. Mama Elena followed behind them, fighting grief and the numbness of shock. When she entered the house, the rooms seemed unbearably silent. The servants were quiet with sorrow after learning of the tragedy. Within the hour Topio returned home empty-handed, devastated by his brother Domingo's death. Domingo—young, handsome, intelligent, and kind—had been the family's favorite. But Mama Elena could not think of Domingo now. She faced the painful task of going next door to Jose Maria's hacienda and informing Sabina. Surely her son's wife would want to accompany her to Mazatlan.

Elena's thoughts were interrupted by a knock on the door. A servant answered and returned moments later, her face ashen. "It is the old man, Maria's father!" she announced in disbelief.

Elena and her visitor exchanged somber greetings.

"I am on my way to Mazatlan to be with my son," he told her, fidgeting nervously with the *sombrero* in his hands. "But I had to see you first. I—I suffer with you over the loss of Domingo. My Maria loved him so. And I loved him like a son."

"You did not have to come here to tell me that," replied Elena.

"But I did," persisted the man. "Lenita, I wish Juan had killed me and not Domingo. Juan was never a worthwhile citizen. He was devious. He turned my other sons into rebellious, impetuous fellows." He paused, groping for words. "There is something you should know, Lenita.

Juan . . . was not my son. He was my servant. I adopted him long ago, before I had children of my own. Even Maria and my true sons do not know this. Only Juan knew."

"That is why he hated Domingo?" questioned Elena incredulously.

"Yes. He was crazy with jealousy. Juan wanted Maria for himself."

Elena turned toward the fireplace, trembling slightly as she straightened her shoulders. "Thank you for telling me."

"There is one more thing, Lenita." The man's voice broke slightly. "My son and his friends plan to ambush your son Marciano tonight."

"How do you know?" Elena asked carefully, her voice controlled.

"I heard them talking. They have shotguns. They know the route Marciano travels. They plan to riddle him with bullets as he rides by."

Elena swiveled slowly, still not looking at her guest. "Why are you telling me this?"

"Maria and I want no more bloodshed," the father replied simply.

"Nor I." Elena remained motionless for several minutes until she heard footsteps on the tile and the large paneled front door closed behind the old man. Then she turned resolutely to her servant. "Saddle me a horse," she said. "Now!"

SIX

The moon shone bleakly on a lone woman riding horseback across the desert.

Several servants had insisted on accompanying Mama Elena, but she had refused. Marciano would be suspicious if he were met by so many. Who would notice a single rider in the evening shadows? Better that she go alone.

In her mind she rehearsed what she would say to Marciano. No mention of this noon's tragedy, no word about the ambushers who lay in wait. Chano would be overwhelmed with anger if he knew the truth; he would confront his enemies and there would be more violence.

When she spotted Marciano and his *mozos* galloping over the tundra toward her, Elena waved and forced a cheerful greeting.

Marciano was pleased but puzzled to see her. "Mama Elena, why do you ride out at evening to meet me?"

"A business matter, my son," she replied briskly. "I want you to take another route home with me to inspect a parcel of land I may wish to purchase."

"But why now—when it is so late in the day?"

"To save you an extra journey, Chano," she explained.

Several hours later they arrived home, without incident, safe. Not until they were inside the protective walls of the main house did Elena dare to reveal the crushing news.

Marciano wept bitterly. "If only you had allowed me to face my attackers! I would have claimed their lives for Domingo's sake!"

The following morning the Hernandez family traveled to Mazatlan. At the hospital they learned that Jose Maria had undergone surgery. His condition remained critical, but the doctors gave him a slim chance of survival. Over the next few weeks he improved steadily.

During his convalescence, Jose Maria was placed under house arrest for murder. When he was finally released from the hospital, the authorities took him immediately to jail.

Determined to prevent a long prison term for her son, Mama Elena insisted on a private hearing with the judge. "I have much wealth, but it does me no good if my son wastes his life in jail," she told the magistrate. "I would give much to secure my son's freedom."

The judge's expression remained stoical, but his eyes gleamed and he massaged his knuckles greedily. "Perhaps something can be arranged, Sra. Hernandez. But I will not allow your son to return to Villa Unión. There would undoubtedly be more killings. Hatred and vengeance would eventually destroy both families."

"Then what can we do?"

"If I release Jose Maria, you and your family must liquidate all your properties and possessions and leave Mexico. You must sever all ties and never return."

"Leave Mexico?"

"It is the only way to prevent reprisals."

"But our home . . . and all that we have worked to build—"

"It is your choice, Sra. Hernandez."

There was really no choice for Elena. Prepared to do whatever was necessary to save her son, she accepted the judge's condition and paid the exorbitant amount he demanded.

After Jose Maria's release, he went into hiding, spending the next several months regaining his strength at the family ranch in distant Hermosillo while his family prepared to leave Villa Unión.

One day Elena and Marciano arrived in Hermosillo with

news for Jose Maria: they were ready to cross the border into Arizona.

"Chema, are you feeling well enough to travel?" quizzed Marciano, greeting his brother with an embrace.

"I am like a new man," replied Jose Maria, flexing an arm muscle in jest. "But I go crazy with nothing to do in this place."

"In Arizona there will be much to do," said Mama Elena. "You and Chano must find work and establish homes in Nogales. I will accompany you. Then I will return to Villa Unión to complete negotiations for our properties. In a few weeks I will escort your sisters and your wives and children to Arizona."

"Will none of the family remain in Mexico?" asked Jose Maria.

"Only your first cousin Gregorio Navarro and his family."

"Ah, yes, our *Cacurrichi*—he is quiet and humble and hard-working. He will have no trouble." Jose Maria gripped his mother affectionately by the shoulders. "Tell me, Mama, how is Sabina and Jose Jr. and my new little daughter Elena?"

"They are well, Chema. Eager to be with you again."

"I am eager too." He gestured toward a table spread with food. "I am forgetting my manners. Come. Eat. We have plenty of tortillas, *frijoles* and *chicharon*—crisp pork fat."

As they ate, they talked nostalgically about the past and the life they would be leaving behind.

"We go not to the United States by choice," admitted Jose Maria reluctantly. "Does it grieve you greatly, Mama, to leave our homeland?"

"I grieve some," she confessed, "but mainly I remember. I think of your papa and of my own mama and papa."

"Revolutionaries, your mama and papa!" noted Marciano teasingly.

"No, Chano. Mexican social reformers," snapped Elena.

"*Mexican*? Grandfather Mácimo was Italian and Grandmother Irinéa a beautiful French lady and a '*doctora partera*'—a midwife."

"Yes. Irinéa Aldaco was a respected, well-educated woman," recalled Elena proudly.

"But, of course, there was their son Sostenes," remarked Marciano, casting a shrewd glance at his brother.

"Sostenes was not their son," growled Jose Maria. "I will never consider him part of our family."

"But he was indeed Grandfather Mácimo's son—his child by the family maid. It is the truth. Why should we deny it?"

"Enough, Chano," insisted Mama Elena.

Marciano frowned. "But Sostenes is your very own half-brother, Mama."

"He should not have been. Mama Irinéa never knew. I did not know until after Papa died. It was a well-guarded family secret."

Elena stood up from the table and walked over to the window. "My Mama Irinéa had a maid she liked very much. This maid became pregnant and had no husband, so my father suggested that he and Mama keep the child. Sostenes was raised as my adopted brother." Elena gazed reflectively out the window. "I remember my father telling me, 'Take care of this boy, Elena. Take good care of him. Later on you will know why I am telling you these words.'"

"But what about the locket your father gave you?" questioned Marciano.

"My father gave me the '*escapulario*' and told me not to open it until after his death. Of course I obeyed his word."

"The locket contained a message—"

"Yes. It said, 'Elena, my daughter, forgive me. Sostenes is your half-brother, your own flesh. Treat him kindly.'" She paused, then added quietly, "When Sostenes learned the truth, he felt great shame."

"Where is Sostenes now?"

"In Puerto Vallarta. We no longer have contact with him."

"It is just as well," snapped Jose Maria. "I will never consider Sostenes my uncle!"

"Perhaps we should talk about something more agreeable," suggested Elena, returning to the table.

"Yes," said Marciano, nodding. "Tell us about you and Papa."

"Ah, your papa . . . my Benceslau. Such a man he was. So tall and strong and clever, with the most handsome green eyes." Elena smiled, remembering. "When Benceslau came to Villa Unión, he had no money, but he possessed great wisdom and ambition. He succeeded at everything he tried. Over the years he accumulated warehouses and lands, his crops flourished, and his cattle grew fat. We always had many visitors in our home, and many good times."

"He should not have died so soon," murmured Jose Maria ruefully. "Such a freak accident—our papa thrown by that crazy burro."

Mama Elena looked up sadly. "I remember thinking he had recovered from the fall. He seemed better."

"I recall the night he died," said Marciano. "Papa was talking to you and Chema and me. He said he felt tired and was going to bed early."

"He had a fever," added Elena, "but he didn't complain. He kept advising me about the business operations and our financial commitments. I couldn't understand why." Elena's voice grew tremulous. "I said to him, 'You stop talking like that, Benceslau. You will see to it that we never have to worry about financial matters, so stop joking.' Then I helped him to bed and went to the kitchen to fix him some soup. When I returned to his room, I found him dead."

Elena brushed at her eyes and glanced away. "Look at us," she scoffed. "We were going to talk about *pleasant* things!"

Marciano patted his mother's hand and smiled. "We could talk about the time you threw the heavy clay pot at me."

Jose Maria laughed impulsively. "I remember that. You always hated household chores, Chano. You came in the house carrying a pail of water and said, 'Well, where do you want the water?'"

"It was a silly question," clucked Elena. "I replied sarcastically, 'How about anywhere you wish!'"

"So I dumped the pail on the floor at Mama's feet," said Marciano.

Elena smiled in amusement, her eyes still glistening with unshed tears. "So I picked up the nearest heavy object and flung it at you as you leaped out the window."

"I never complained about chores again!"

"You didn't dare," chuckled Jose Maria. "Mama had an inexhaustible supply of clay pots!" They laughed heartily.

Then Mama Elena and her sons grew silent, relishing the unexpected closeness of the moment.

"Papa would be proud of you, Mama Elena," said Marciano earnestly. "Nothing bends you or breaks you; your children look to you for strength."

Elena straightened her back and set her chin determinedly. "My greatest challenge faces me tomorrow—delivering my sons swiftly into Arizona, then bringing your families safely from Villa Unión."

"It will go well," said Marciano reassuringly. "We will be settled in the United States before we know it."

Jose Maria's expression sobered. "And I will count the days until I am able to return to Mexico."

Elena stared in astonishment at her son. "No, Chema! We can never return to Mexico. That was the agreement for your freedom."

"You agreed, Mama Elena, not I. Mexico will always be my home. Someday, when the trouble has been forgotten, I will return."

SEVEN

In September 1922 the Hernandez family settled in the United States and began to work on a ranch near Scottsdale, Arizona. While Jose Maria worked the fields, Marciano peddled vegetables in a little truck to neighboring ranches.

After a few months, Jose Maria's wife Sabina announced that she was pregnant with their third child. Immediately Jose made plans to return to Mexico. No one—nothing— could convince him to stay.

"My sons and daughters must be Mexicans," he said vehemently.

"But it is not safe to return to Villa Unión," argued Mama Elena.

"We will go to Santiago Ixcuintla in the state of Nayarit," he told her. "We have distant relatives there who will help us."

"But is it wise for Sabina to travel so far in her condition?"

Jose Maria gazed severely at his mother. "It is already settled, Mama Elena. My heart is in Mexico."

As Jose Maria wished, his daughter Jessie, or Chuy, was born in Mexico. But promptly after her birth, Jose Maria, suspecting trouble, moved his family back to the States, near Phoenix. The children that followed— Apolonia, Ester, Benceslau, Rosario, Alejandro, Leonardo, Eloisa, Ricardo, Ruby, and Lila—were born in the United States.

On Jose Maria's return, he and his brother Marciano became farm laborers on the ranch of an Italian named Cruz. Jose, who in Mexico had been a supervisor accustomed to affluence and power, found field work back-breaking toil offering little financial remuneration. He realized with a dismaying jolt that since leaving Mexico, he had nothing . . . *was* nothing.

Then a chance encounter with a shrewd, sinister man named Angel Morales altered the direction of Jose Maria's life. Morales, a highly successful liquor smuggler, was rich, suave, confident, and immaculately dressed—everything Jose Maria wished desperately to be.

"We could use you in our operation," observed Morales after Jose had talked at some length about his life in Mexico.

"What would you have me do?" questioned Jose Maria.

"Make liquor for us," replied Morales. "During these days of Prohibition, bootlegging is extremely profitable in this country."

"But I would need equipment, a place to work."

"I understand your ranch is nicely isolated . . ."

Jose Maria shook his head doubtfully. "I have a cellar, but I live on Sr. Cruz's ranch. He might become suspicious."

"The main house is some distance from your ranch, isn't it?" said Morales. "I assure you, precautions can be taken to prevent detection." His lips curled into a sneering grin. "We ship our liquor into many states. You would become a wealthy man, Sr. Hernandez."

Jose Maria quickly returned the smile. "Wealthy, you say? Then you have found your man, Sr. Morales."

They spent the rest of the day making arrangements and inspecting Jose Maria's ranch to determine what would be required to transform the cellar into a liquor factory and warehouse. When Sr. Morales learned that Jose Maria's mother and sisters Jovita and Victoria occupied another ranch on the Cruz property, he suggested establishing distilleries at both houses.

"This will be no small business venture," Morales stressed. "I will provide the equipment and stock, including sugar and yeast, and peaches, prunes, and raisins for flavoring. I'll buy all the liquor you can produce."

Three stills, made of copper, were eventually constructed. Sr. Morales instructed Jose Maria, and later Marciano, in processing the liquor. "Every barrel of fermentation will produce from two to ten gallons of whiskey," explained Morales. "For every fifty gallons of water, you will need sixty pounds of sugar and about three pounds of yeast to ferment the water."

"It will be a miracle if Cruz does not discover our operation," mused Jose Maria.

"It is your responsibility to see that he detects nothing," warned Sr. Morales. "Once the authorities suspect you, they will hound you mercilessly."

"They will learn nothing from me," Jose Maria assured him firmly.

"You will need many truckloads of wood to maintain the temperature of the fermented solution," continued Morales. "But keep in mind, a fire too hot or too cool will ruin the whiskey."

"I will manage," replied Jose Maria. "You forget that I made liquor in Mexico."

"But never on so grand a scale," returned the man cunningly.

Once the distilleries were in operation, Angel Morales arrived once every fifteen days, around midnight, in an expensive Dodge truck. Five hundred gallons of liquor in twenty-gallon barrels were swiftly loaded into the bed of the truck and hidden beneath a specially made covering, for transport to New Mexico and other adjoining states.

The system worked smoothly for many months. By day Jose Maria labored in the fields for Sr. Cruz; at night he ran the stills. It was a grinding schedule, but Jose Maria thrived. He was in control, managing his own life, and in time would accumulate a tidy fortune. Money was power . . . and power was everything!

Then early one evening, police officers pulled up in front of the Hernandez ranch, stepped out of their automobile, and strode toward Jose Maria. He greeted the visitors with feigned cheerfulness. But his smile sagged when one officer said bluntly, "Hernandez, word is out you got a bootleggin' business goin' on here."

"You are mistaken, señor," said Jose Maria.

"Then you won't mind us lookin' around," snorted the policeman.

Before Jose Maria could reply, the officers took long sticks with half-inch knives on the ends and began poking the ground, probing for buried whiskey barrels.

Minutes later there was the telltale thud of a blade striking wood. "Looks like we got one here," one officer told the other. The men looked at Jose Maria. "You better go tell your missus you're leavin' for a spell, Mr. Hernandez. You're under arrest for bootleggin'."

For Jose Maria it would be the first of twenty-one arrests for manufacturing illegal whiskey. But spending a few days in jail didn't faze him. After each release, he resumed his liquor operation with the passion and vigor of a man returning from a dull vacation to the job he loves. But Jose Maria cherished more than his work and the money he made. He craved the liquor—and lately was drinking increasingly greater amounts. And why not? It was there, free, plentiful. Why hadn't he realized before that it was liquor that helped him face the pressures every day?

Often Angel Morales visited Jose Maria with ideas for improving their operation. He originated a method for "painting" the liquor a deep cherry red by using burnt sugar. Eventually Morales streamlined his color processing system by evenly burning the insides of the liquor barrels to produce an expensive, unique liquor called "*añiejo*."

Another time Morales studied the distilling equipment and said with deliberation, "How much wood are you burning each week?"

"One or two *cuerdas*," replied Jose Maria.

"That's a lot of wood," said Morales. "What would you think of switching to butane burners? Butane would make it easier to regulate the temperature."

"I'm for anything that makes the job easier or brings in more cash," replied Jose Maria.

But as Jose Maria gained confidence and proficiency in manufacturing liquor, he decided he wanted to call the shots himself, be his own boss. So eventually he and Morales parted company. Jose Maria reigned alone as king of the bootleg ring, one of the largest such undertakings ever to operate in Arizona.

As Jose Maria's wealth and influence grew, his life took on powerful new facets. He had always been a man of impressive contradictions; now more than ever he straddled two extreme life-styles. He was an indomitable underworld figure surrounded by doting admirers from the Mexican and Puerto Rican communities, and a reclusive, short-tempered man dauntlessly pursued by the authorities and incapacitated, even possessed, by alcohol.

To the world at large, he was a man to be feared and respected; at least he saw himself that way. His reputation had spread widely, and he had accumulated many friends. Lovely young ladies noticed him and flirted coyly. Although Jose Maria stood only 5' 7", he was solid, even brawny, and had handsome, chiseled features. He did not find it surprising that women considered him attractive. He found them equally appealing and made new conquests as he pleased. Wherever he went, he spent his money freely.

Wishing to enhance his image, Jose Maria began to wear a white suit and an expensive straw hat. He carried a cane he did not need and was always armed with a gun. He became such a legend in Phoenix that acquaintances wrote ballads, or *corridos*, about him. Several Puerto Rican friends, who sought Jose Maria's friendship by introducing him to available women, wrote a special *corrido* and sang it for him, using pots, plates, forks and spoons as instruments.

Levantate Chema, Levantate Chema,
que los que te cantan de Puerto Rico son.
Get up, Chema, get up, Chema.
Those of us who sing to you are from Puerto Rico.

While Jose Maria was lauded and applauded by his companions, he became a figure of fear and contempt at home. His wife, Sabina, bruised both in spirit and body by his philandering and his drunken rages, had grown to despise him. Still, scrupulously faithful to the ingrained Mexican tradition of *machismo*, or male supremacy, Sabina silently and obediently served her husband, met his needs, and reared his children. His command was law, his authority unquestioned.

Jose Maria was a man of few words: You go . . . You stay . . . You arrive at this hour. When he said, "Everyone to bed," the family promptly retired; when he said, "Everyone up for work," they scrambled out of their beds.

The older Hernandez youngsters were subjected to frequent beatings for even minor infractions, and were forced to labor long hours in the distilleries. They made routine trips to the jail to pay bail to secure their father's release. And they suffered in agonized silence when, from time to time, their father viciously lashed their mother. On one occasion Jose Maria chased Sabina through the house with a machete. Another time, enraged over some supposed wrongdoing, he drew his gun and fired a shot at his wife, miraculously just missing her. Then twelve-year-old Jose Jr. watched in horror as his father grabbed Sabina by the hair and dragged her several feet. When he finally cast her down, he still clutched strands of her hair in his hand.

In his own mind, Jose Maria was simply exercising his rights as head of his household. Didn't his family exist for his pleasure, his convenience? He envisioned himself as someone invincible, insulated by his money and prestige. All Phoenix knew of his influence and power; even local police and governmental authorities could not deter him. No one dared cross Don Jose Maria Hernandez!

Jose Maria might have been less arrogant had he foreseen that shortly a series of bizarre, unrelated incidents would carry him on a downward spiral into stabbing poverty, self-loathing, and overwhelming despair, from which only God himself could deliver him. But for the moment he was blithely, heedlessly riding the crest of pomp and prosperity.

EIGHT

While Jose Maria thrived on his success as a bootlegger, his older brother Marciano and his grown sisters Jovita and Victoria looked elsewhere for meaning in life. They turned to the church.

Their search for faith began with Marciano who, hungry for spiritual truths, started attending an Adventist church. He invited the rest of the family, but everyone refused. Finally Jovita and Victoria attended twice, only for Chano's sake.

Then one weekend as the two Hernandez sisters walked along Washington Street in Phoenix, they passed a Pentacostal minister preaching on a street corner. Loudly he exclaimed, "One day we may search for God, but we won't find him!"

For several days the thought pressed ominously on Jovita's mind: *One day I may search for God and not find him.*

Months later Mama Elena, Jovita, and Victoria returned to Mexico to attend to some unfinished family business. Jovita, a devoted Catholic, was astonished to discover that the churches in Mexico had been closed because of a recent revolution. Despair engulfed her as she stood before the bolted doors of a deserted cathedral. She felt as if God had been locked away from her forever. After all, wasn't God found only in church? Now the accessible God was beyond reach. The words of the Pentecostal preacher thundered in her consciousness and filled her with nightmarish horror. Weeping unashamedly, she said over and over, "God has left us. He has left me! I'll never find him again!"

One day after their return to Phoenix, Jovita invited Victoria and her two cousins to join her at a little Baptist church nearby to make fun of the "*Protestantes*." Brother Leonardo Mercado, a large man with a broad face and small, twinkling eyes, was preaching on the subject, "What shall it profit a man if he gain the whole world and lose his own soul?" Immediately the haunting words of the Pentecostal preacher came back to Jovita. She had come here to poke fun and ridicule; instead, she was hearing the same disquieting warning.

As the congregation began to sing "The Old Rugged Cross," Jovita's eyes filled with tears. She felt as if something within her would explode. She slipped out of the sanctuary, rushed to the bathroom, and sobbed uncontrollably. Her heart pounded and she felt short of breath. God was speaking to her in a startling new way. Drying her eyes, she returned for the conclusion of the service. No sooner had she sat down than Brother Mercado invited people to repent of their sins and give their lives to the Lord Jesus Christ. For Jovita, it was an eternity to the altar, but resolutely she made her way forward. She later described her conversion as "such a beautifully rich experience that I thought I had one foot inside Heaven."

When Jovita shared her experience with Mama Elena, adding that she planned to be baptized in the Baptist church, Elena Hernandez was outraged. "How dare you forsake our church! And you call yourself my daughter! How can I be the mother of one such as you?"

With trembling voice, Jovita replied, "Kill me if you must . . . if what I've done offends you. But don't tell me you will cease being my mother. I must obey God. I hope someday to see you also commit your life to the Lord Jesus."

"I do not wish to discuss such things with you," growled Mama Elena.

"Is it because you would have to stop selling liquor for Chema?"

"What do you mean?" demanded Elena.

"Since we moved here to Tenth Street in Phoenix, you have made your living smuggling and selling Chema's whiskey," said Jovita. "I know that is why people come here at all hours of the day or night."

"I have not tried to hide it from you," Elena remarked defensively.

"But it is wrong!" cried Jovita.

"Hush," said Elena. "It is my livelihood—and Chema's." Her eyes narrowed disapprovingly. "Do not let your brother know that you have forsaken our church. He is the church's most stalwart defender."

"Ha!" clucked Jovita. "Jose Maria refuses even to enter the church. Do you remember the time in Mexico when you asked him to accompany me to Mass? He said, 'No, you will never see me hanging around a bunch of old ladies!' "

"And I slapped him hard for that," returned Mama Elena.

"He is too old and too powerful now to slap," reflected Jovita. "But I pray with all my heart for him . . . and for you, Mama Elena."

Jovita's sister Victoria was the second member of the Hernandez family to yield her life to the Lord. Then came Marciano, eager and rejoicing. Following his conversion, Marciano left the bootlegging business, explaining, "I do not wish to break Christian laws." He bought a truck and went from ranch to ranch, selling merchandise to the cotton-pickers. He was so successful as a businessman that eventually he was able to buy a lot on Seventh Avenue in Phoenix and build a store. In time, he purchased almost an entire city block on Seventh Avenue, and still later he would return to Mazatlan and then Hermosillo, Mexico, to open his own business.

Not long after her conversion, Jovita married a man named Jose who showed little patience with her faith or her attachment to Brother Mercado's church. One evening as she prepared to leave for prayer meeting, Jose told her, "We have come to the crossroad. You must choose between your God and me. If you go now to church, do not return to my house."

Jovita stood momentarily silent. In her heart she knew she could never abandon her commitment to Christ. Picking up her purse and jewelry, she went outside, climbed into her little Model-T sedan, and headed for church. She felt nervous, distraught, wondering whether she was doing the right thing. Surely she wanted to obey God, but didn't she also have a sacred responsibility to her husband?

Jovita found some comfort in sitting with her brother Marciano in church. But early in the service she noticed her husband looking in through the side window. Her heart leaped in fear. In the past Jose had threatened to burst in and drag her out of church. Would he cause such a disturbance now?

Jovita heard little of the message, even though, halfway through, her husband apparently went home. After the service, Jovita drove straight to her mother's house.

"What has happened?" Mama Elena asked anxiously at the door.

"Well, you see, Jose had to work tonight," stammered Jovita, "and I didn't want to be alone . . . so here I am." It was a lie, of course, but Jovita refused to complain to her family about her husband's contrary behavior.

The next day Jovita drove, as usual, to a residence where she worked as a housekeeper. When she returned to her car that afternoon, she found her husband sitting in the driver's seat, waiting for her.

Quelling her misgivings, Jovita asked him to unlock the door and move over. He moved without a word. Jovita slipped inside, started the engine, and began to drive to her mother's house.

"Where are you going?" asked Jose. "You just passed our home!"

"No," said Jovita simply. "You said I didn't have a home with you if I attended church."

"Can't we talk about it?" questioned Jose. "I want to know your intentions."

"I plan to serve God."

Her husband's voice quavered slightly. "Forgive me, Jovita, for being so hotheaded. You see, I don't quite understand these things. I promise never again to prohibit your attending church."

Jovita gazed at her husband with a grateful smile. "Then I

am happy to resume our marriage. I am glad I can love my God and love you too."

That evening when Jovita returned from Bible study at Brother Mercado's, her husband greeted her with freshly baked biscuits and hot coffee. He never harassed her again.

Jovita's husband was a kind, simple man, but over the years he became an alcoholic. Whenever she invited him to join her at church, he would inevitably reply, "I can't stop drinking, Jovita. I'm sorry, but I won't play games with God. I will take the step when I think I can keep my promise to him."

Some time later, Jovita's husband was struck and killed by an automobile. She felt the loss deeply. Shortly before the funeral, her pastor found her crying disconsolately.

" Sister Jovita, be of good cheer," he told her. "Your husband is in Heaven in the presence of the Lord!"

Jovita looked up stunned. "But he never accepted the Lord."

"That's what I want to share with you," replied the minister eagerly. "Five days before the accident, your husband came to visit me. He wept and said he regretted the suffering he had caused you. We prayed together and he gave his life to Christ. Didn't he tell you?"

"No," cried Jovita, mingling tears of joy with those of grief. "I didn't know!"

While Jovita, Victoria, and Marciano served God faithfully at Brother Mercado's Baptist church, Jose Maria became increasingly infuriated over their involvement in the religion of the *Protestantes*. Distressingly for Jose Maria, the conflict touched closer home, within his own household.

He had recently moved his family to the "Golden Gate" district of Phoenix to evade the authorities. Here in Golden Gate his family had begun attending the Episcopalian church, the only house of worship in the neighborhood. Jose Maria had permitted their attendance at first, assuming that the church was simply an Americanized version of the Catholic church in Mexico. The cleric robes were similar and from what he had heard, the liturgy and worship ceremonies were nearly the same. Jose Maria even allowed his family to join the church, and Jose Jr. became an altar boy, assisting in Communion services. But when the rector distributed Bibles to each member, Jose Maria, horrified at such an unseemly deed, forcibly prohibited his family from further attendance at the Episcopal church.

But other, more pressing matters were plaguing Jose Maria now. A fire in the distillery at the ranch—and more recently a conflagration in their cellar at Golden Gate—had destroyed much of Jose Maria's distilling equipment. Replacement was costly. Worse, Jose Maria was under constant surveillance these days. Whenever he attempted to reestablish his bootlegging operation, the authorities appeared, confiscated his equipment, and hauled him off to jail. Release fees were mounting.

To complicate the situation still further, governmental agencies were seeking any reason whatever to deport Jose Maria to Mexico. They considered him an undesirable alien. In the past, Sr. Cruz had handled all immigration matters. Without Cruz as an intermediary, Jose Maria found himself hounded incessantly by the immigration service.

It frustrated Jose Maria that the glamor of his life-style was growing dim, the excitement degenerating into unrelenting tension. Lately, no matter how much liquor he drank, the pressures and problems remained.

One day there was another police raid. Jose Maria and his distilling equipment were loaded on the back of a truck and paraded through the main streets of Phoenix, with police escorts forming an unlikely caravan. People stopped and stared curiously as the peculiar exhibition trundled through town. Children ran beside the truck, shouting. Dogs barked. Old men and women peered down from second-story windows. Jose Maria sat bound to his equipment, a public spectacle.

"We want the people of this city to see just what you've been doing," an officer told Jose Maria. "You're no big shot, mister, just a common criminal!"

Jose Maria ground his jaw with loathing and spat on the ground. "If you think you can shame me, you are all fools," he said, laughing scornfully. "No one shames Don Jose Maria Hernandez!"

A week later, the incident was nearly forgotten as Jose Maria kept a romantic tryst with an attractive young woman whose husband was away on business. The two met often, and Jose felt much affection for the woman. The following evening he encountered her again, unexpectedly, at a party. She was with her husband, a stuffy, unpleasant fellow named Fimbres. Jose was jealous, on edge, at seeing the two together, but he managed polite indifference when the couple greeted him. Jose and the man drank and exchanged small talk for a while in a private corner of the house. Somehow, as the whiskey flowed, a word slipped out inadvertently, and Fimbres caught a lingering glance between Jose and his wife. Without warning, Fimbres grew quarrelsome and loudly vented his suspicions. "So it is you, Jose Maria. You are my wife's lover!"

As the man raved, Jose impulsively drew his gun and fired. The bullet exploded through the man's leg.

Fimbres collapsed, moaning, "You'll pay, Hernandez. You'll pay!"

Jose Maria recognized the terrible truth of the man's words. As party guests rushed into the room, Jose shouted, "Get a doctor. This man was accidentally shot!"

Bending over Fimbres, Jose Maria whispered urgently, "Don't report me, please! I'll take care of your medical expenses. I'll pay whatever you ask."

Fimbres managed a nod. In the days that followed, Jose Maria paid liberally for the man's silence.

NINE

Late one night in 1934, not long after shooting Fimbres, Jose
Maria awoke to find the room filled with dense smoke. "*Ay
de mi!*" he cried. "The distilling equipment is on fire again!"
He jumped up coughing, shouting. "Sabina! Jose! Chuy!
Apolonia!"

He ran from one room to another, rousing his family
while flames licked the walls, leaping across curtains,
tables, and chairs. Streams of fire erupted from the cellar and
swept over the floor in jagged lightning streaks.

"*Vamonos!* Everyone out!" rasped Jose Maria, shielding
his face from the fumes. Minutes later the Hernandez family
huddled together in their yard, watching helplessly as their
house burned to the ground.

The next morning they inspected the devastation. Tears
mixed with grime and soot on Sabina's face as she sobbed,
"Everything is gone. We have lost everything!"

"The liquor fed the flames," observed her fifteen-year-old
son Jose.

Jose Maria shook his head in disbelief. "All my money,
gone," he groaned. "Thousands of dollars in the mattress
burned to ashes." He stooped down and picked up a
shapeless, hardened mass of metal. "And all my coins
melted."

Jose, Jr. embraced his mother in a futile gesture of

comfort. "Papa never should have left his money all over the house in those old tin cans."

Sabina nodded ruefully. "He does not believe in banks. He always said he would never do business with them."

Jose Maria straightened his shoulders and set his jaw. "Do not fret yourselves," he said. "I have friends. They will help me get started in business again."

But Jose Maria was gravely mistaken. Without his wealth, he no longer had friends. Conveniently forgotten were the *corridos*, the flamboyant legends, the good times. He was a bankrupt man; his admirers had scattered.

Stubbornly refusing to admit defeat, Jose Maria moved his family into a modest home, still in the Golden Gate district of Phoenix, and went out looking for a job. There would be no more bootlegging, but business had been faltering anyway since the repeal of the Prohibition law the year before.

"So what if I have to start over, make it on my own?" he told his family with forced optimism. "I'll show everyone what I can do. As long as I can work, we will survive." He began making adobes—baked straw and mud blocks—to sell to building contractors, and helped cut wood in his brother Marciano's lumberyard.

One evening there was a knock on Jose Maria's door. When he opened it, a strapping man well over six feet tall greeted him with a generous smile. "I am Brother Leonardo Mercado from the Iglesia Evangelica," he said. "I would like to invite you and your family to our Baptist church."

Jose Maria stared up at the man in mute surprise. After a moment he said, "Is that the church my brother Chano and my sisters attend?"

"Yes," said the minister. "And we are pleased that recently your mother, Elena Hernandez, became a Christian and was baptized."

"And now you would have my children become 'hallelu-jahs' too!" barked Jose Maria.

"And you also, Sr. Hernandez."

In an impulsive gesture of disgust, Jose Maria raised his right hand and struck Brother Mercado across the face. The minister flinched momentarily, then steadied himself, and said softly, "Brother Jose Maria, you may slap my other cheek."

Baffled, Jose Maria hesitated, then retreated. Struggling to control his voice, he said, "Leave, señor. I have nothing more to say to you."

Not long after Brother Mercado's visit, Jose Maria was ordered to go to Nogales for clearance to remain in the States. "Those fools! Still they hound me!" he complained to Sabina. "They do not realize I no longer make whiskey. I no longer have influence and power. I am just a poor, hard-working man with many mouths to feed."

In Nogales, the immigration service required Jose Maria to list all his children's names and birth dates in sequence. With alcohol clouding his mind, he could not recall Chuy's full name—Natividad de Jesus. The authorities, looking for any technicality to hold the former bootlegger, and unable to imagine a father forgetting his own child's name, imprisoned him. It appeared that after all his escapades, Jose Maria would be returned to Mexico for the most ludicrous of violations.

In jail, friendless and poverty-stricken, Jose Maria could think of no one to deliver him from his dilemma . . . except Brother Mercado. The minister, well-established in the community, had much influence with local and state authorities. It was known that he had acquired the release of converted prisoners, often assuming full custody of released convicts.

"I want to see Brother Leonardo Mercado," Jose Maria told the authorities.

Within three days Brother Mercado secured Chuy's certificate of baptism containing her full name and birth date, and obtained Jose Maria's release. Out of grudging appreciation, Jose Maria permitted his family to attend Brother Mercado's church from time to time. While he adamantly refused to join them, on occasion, out of curiosity, he asked his wife Sabina to read to him from the Bible.

One morning in 1935, an incident occurred which would change forever the course of Jose Maria's life. He and his son, Jose, Jr. had just arrived for work in Marciano's lumberyard. Activating the makeshift power saw, Jose Maria maneuvered a large piece of timber toward the forbidding blade, three feet in diameter. Suddenly the lumber slipped and Jose Maria's body lurched forward involuntarily. As he thrust out his arm to protect himself, his hand was instantly shattered by the blade. He uttered an oath of horror as blood spurted uncontrollably.

Marciano sprang forward and wrapped a handkerchief around his brother's wound while Jose, Jr. found a piece of wire and secured the crude temporary bandage. They gathered fragments of the hand in a paper bag, then rushed Jose Maria to the hospital.

Several hours later, a stony-faced doctor met with Marciano and Jose, Jr. and explained, "We were not able to restore the hand. We amputated just above the wrist. It was a matter of saving his life."

Jose Maria remained in the hospital for a week and was fitted for a gloved prosthesis for his wrist and hand. Then he was sent home.

A man in shock—that was Jose Maria. In the months that followed, he became a recluse—somber, remote, introspective. He saw himself as half a man, a cripple, brutally emasculated, stripped of pride, vigor, and independence. He could no longer work. He was forced to relearn even the simplest routine tasks. For many months he suffered relentless pain and struggled to adjust to the grim "phantom hand syndrome."

As the permanence of his condition gripped him, Jose Maria sank into a morass of depression. Convinced that he had become an object of ridicule, he sat in his house and brooded, refusing to go out in public.

Over and over the question plagued him: Why did he have to lose his hand? And why his right hand, his best hand! One day a curious thought dawned. That was the hand he had used to slap Brother Mercado, a man of God. And the hand with which he had committed murder and near murder. Perhaps God was punishing him for those transgressions. What did they call it—retribution? If that were the case, reflected Jose Maria, then he owed much more than a hand. He had committed so many evil deeds in his lifetime; surely he owed his arms, his legs, all that he had. *All would not be enough*. It was a despairing realization.

Slowly, tenaciously, Jose Maria emerged from the clutches of despondency and began to reassert himself. He grew restless, irritable, yearning to work again, to be useful, productive. Often he paced the floor, lamenting, "What can I do! These days even healthy men cannot find work. Who will hire a bankrupt, uneducated immigrant with a prison record . . . and only one hand!"

The burden of providing for the entire Hernandez household lay oppresively now on Jose, Jr., a sixteen-year-old with only a third-grade education. Early every morning the youth trekked to the market with a little wagon to search among the trash barrels for discarded, overripe fruit and vegetables. He collected stale bread and pastries from the bakeries, routinely removing mold and mildew, and gathered wild spinach along the railroad tracks. He scavenged behind the meat stores and packing companies, seizing bones with bits of meat, often soiled with sawdust, and pig's feet or a pig's head to boil in water for soup.

Jose, Jr. eventually found work in the fields. For a negligible fee, he and his father hauled workers back and forth in a small truck. Jose, Jr. sold fruit, soft drinks, and *tortillas* at lunchtime. Later he would actually supervise the workers. He earned eight cents an hour and worked ten hours a day. He did not mind hard work. In fact, he found a certain dignity and satisfaction in earning a living, providing for his parents and younger brothers and sisters. As his self-confidence grew, he sensed he could manage whatever life threw at him. One way or another, he would survive.

Brother Mercado's Baptist church was another source of satisfaction for Jose, Jr. He attended often, taking an eager part in the young people's activities. Many of his relatives were members now.

Then, one day in May 1936, Jose's father, his face reddening with fury, confronted him and demanded, "What is this I have heard about you being baptized in Brother Mercado's church?"

The lean, swarthy youth nodded. "It is true. I accepted Jesus three months ago. And on Easter Sunday I was baptized."

"I never should have allowed you to step foot inside that church," stormed Jose Maria. He gripped his son's shoulder with his one good hand and sent him sprawling against the wall. He struck him repeatedly, then bellowed, "If you have joined the *Protestantes*, get out of my house!"

Hearing the commotion, Sabina rushed into the room. When she saw her son lying bruised and dazed, she cried out in alarm.

"I'm sorry, Mama. Papa says I must leave because I joined the Baptist church," Jose told her as she helped him to his feet. "I will go to live in Uncle Chano's house."

A week later a subdued Jose Maria visited his brother Marciano's home and in a calm, sober voice asked to see his son. The young man greeted his father reticently.

"I want you to come home," said Jose Maria.

Young Jose's face brightened immediately. "Papa, I will come home gladly," he said.

But Jose Maria found other, more subtle ways to curtail his son's freedom. He imposed restrictive rules (no midweek church activities) and insisted that Jose, Jr. be home from weekend services by nine P.M. He increased Jose's chores at home, confiscated whatever money he earned, and beat him severely for the slightest hint of disobedience.

Jose, Jr. prayed fervently for God's peace in his home. He begged the Lord to touch his father's heart and deliver him from his bitterness. The youth prayed, too, for his own fomenting emotions, that he would not harbor hatred and resentment toward his father.

One day Jose Maria received a visit from Marciano and Mama Elena. They talked for a while about mundane family matters and the hard times the country was facing—the lack of good jobs, the high price of food, the special problems facing minorities.

"Roosevelt's WPA program is helping some," observed Marciano.

"Yes," said Jose Maria. "Between Roosevelt and my son, Jose, Jr., we may yet get back on our feet."

"Tell me, Chema," said Marciano with a smile, "when are you coming to church with us?"

Jose Maria scowled. "What place do I have in church? I am not a religious man."

"Come, Chema," laughed Marciano. "Did you ever consider *me* a religious man?"

"But my life . . . there is nothing in it that would please God," reflected Jose Maria somberly.

"That does not matter," said Mama Elena. "What is important is that you accept Jesus Christ as your Savior."

"Now you talk like your 'hallelujah' preacher," said Jose Maria caustically. "I do not understand this talk of Jesus."

Elena Hernandez appeared absorbed in thought. Then she put her hand on her son's arm and said, "Chema, do you remember when you were in prison in Mexico? I went to the judge and paid for your freedom. I ransomed you, or you would still be in prison today."

"*Verdad*," said Jose Maria. "Never can I repay what you did for me."

"Neither can we repay what God did for us," said Elena.

"What do you mean?"

"I speak of the evil things we do, Chema—the sin that is in our hearts. There is no way we can make things right with God."

Jose Maria stared glumly at his artificial hand. "I know, Mama Elena. A hand is not enough to give . . . nothing is enough."

Elena squeezed her son's arm affectionately. "Chema, no one can earn salvation. That is why God gave his Son to take the punishment we deserve. Jesus paid the price with his own life. You are free to walk out of the prison that keeps your heart—if you repent of your sins and take Christ as your Savior."

A flicker of yearning crossed Jose Maria's face. "How can I understand your words? How can I know they are true?"

"Come with us to Brother Mercado's church," said Marciano. "He will teach you God's Word."

The following Sunday morning, Jose Maria—his shoulders straight, his chin high—walked boldly into Brother Mercado's church and sat down in a front pew. He riveted his eyes to the preacher and listened intently. He was ready to hear the Word of the Lord.

In the fall of 1936, Jose Maria Hernandez publicly professed his faith in Christ. After his conversion, his life changed dramatically. Although he had been one of the country's most profligate bootleggers and an alcoholic for ten years, Jose Maria put liquor completely out of his life. He immersed himself in the Scriptures. Since he could not read, he insisted on his wife Sabina reading to him from the Bible two hours every day. So enamored did he become with God's Word that he rapidly memorized long passages and delved hungrily into concepts of theology.

Within a year Jose Maria began to preach on the streets of Phoenix, the very streets through which he had been paraded as a shameless criminal only a few years before. The same energy and charisma that had once captivated his Puerto Rican admirers now caught the attention of passers-by as he proclaimed the gospel.

But Jose Maria had not lost his fiery spirit nor his imposing sense of authority. One day as he preached on a street corner, he spotted a drunkard teetering toward him. The man began to heckle him. Jose Maria glanced down from the box where he stood and motioned the fellow away, then continued speaking. But the inebriate stepped closer and shouted in a thick, slurred voice, "It's a lie! Everything he says is a lie!"

As the minutes passed, the drunkard grew bolder and more infuriating. Finally Jose Maria, agitated beyond endurance, paused in mid-sentence, raised his Bible, and roared, "*Amigito, si no se calla le voy a dar un Bibliaso!*—Listen, mister, you better keep quiet or I'm going to hit you over the head with this Bible!"

The mortified tippler slunk away in silence while Jose Maria vigorously resumed his fire and brimstone sermon.

PART THREE
JOSE AND MARGARITA HERNANDEZ

TEN

On Mother's Day in 1936, four months before Jose Maria's conversion, the young people of Brother Mercado's church spent the afternoon gathering flowers in a neighbor's garden. That day Jose Maria's seventeen-year-old son Jose, Jr. approached lovely Margarita Peralta and asked her to be his girl. Sagely the young man advised her not to be hasty in her decision. He would give her fifteen days to make up her mind. If she said yes, she would be agreeing not only to be his girl, but also someday his wife.

During the next two weeks, Margarita spent many hours in prayer. She wondered if Jose Hernandez was the man God had chosen for her. He was a plain man, and poor, with baggy pants and scuffed shoes—not dashing like Tony Sosa and others she had dated. But Jose was serious and hard-working and reliable. Margarita recalled the times she had walked to a nearby canyon and prayed among the rocks. She had told the Lord, "Someday, in the future, if you have a man for me . . . I'm not asking for a rich man, I'm not asking for a good-looking man. But please give me a man who's a Christian, who loves you . . . a hard-working man who loves you."

Jose Hernandez surely fit that description.

So when the fifteen days had passed and Jose came for her answer, Margarita said yes.

Jose beamed. "Now I ask you to call me Chemita, my family name, after my father, Chema." More seriously, he said, "It is only fair that you know I have no money of my own. I receive eight cents an hour as a field hand, but my father keeps my earnings. Still, I will begin now to save twenty-five cents each month for an engagement ring."

Fearful of arousing the anger or suspicion of either of their fathers, Jose and Margarita rarely spent time alone together. Thus, their courtship evolved around the church and young people's activities. Occasionally the assistant minister lent Jose his Model-A automobile, so that Jose could drive Margarita home from youth meetings. But the man also shrewdly sent along Jose's younger sister Elena to sit in the rumble seat.

Nevertheless, over the next few months the couple cherished their brief moments of near privacy. They found countless topics to discuss, including the cruel beatings they had suffered at the hands of their fathers.

"I am so used to those whippings, I think nothing of them anymore," remarked Margarita one evening. "But when Papa comes after me, the one thing I do is put my arms up to protect my head."

"Me too," said Jose. "Papa goes to church with us now, but he still rules with an iron hand. I don't mind the cuts and bruises, but I'm sure careful to hide my head." There was a moment of silence, then Jose asked, "Was your father always so ruthless?"

"Oh, yes," replied Margarita. "He has always demanded absolute obedience from me. Even when I was very small, he would ask for a glass of water and I would run to get it. Then after I handed it to him, I always had to kneel before him and cross my arms until he had finished drinking."

"No wonder you hated him."

"Yes, I did hate him, very much . . . until I became a Christian."

"When was that?" asked Jose.

"Two years ago, through a preacher in Tucson named Brother Morales. I lived with his family for a time while I attended school."

"When did you leave school?"

"In 1935. I had just begun my sophomore year. How I regretted leaving!"

"You were fortunate," observed Jose. "I was able to complete only the third grade before I had to go to work to support my family."

"Education is very important to me," reflected Margarita. "I liked competing in school, and I always felt I had to be the best. But it wasn't easy. I had to take my books out into the mesquites and study in secret by the light of a little candle, sometimes until two in the morning. My father wouldn't let me study in the house."

"You were a very determined girl," said Jose.

Margarita smiled wistfully. "If ever I have children of my own, I will do everything I can to see that they receive an education."

In October 1936, Jose and Margarita became officially engaged. He had saved six dollars for a ring which he proudly slipped on her finger. But they told neither family of their impending marriage, nor did they set a date for the wedding.

Then one evening in December, an incident occurred which made both Jose and Margarita realize that the time was rapidly approaching when they must establish their own home separate from their families. They were attending a young people's Christmas party at church—and thoroughly enjoying themselves. Suddenly they realized it was ten o'clock—and Jose was due home by nine! Margarita and Jose quickly piled into an automobile with several other young people and headed home. Minutes later they dropped Jose off, and he ran into the house.

As the driver started to pull away, Margarita cried, "Wait! Don't go." She peered anxiously toward the house. Her heart lurched involuntarily. The flickering light of a kerosene lamp in the window revealed her beloved Chemita being brutally beaten by his father.

There was stunned silence in the car as everyone's eyes focused on the chilling scene. Margarita turned away, heartsick. In mute frustration she realized that the same fate awaited her at home.

"Why does he accept such treatment?" asked someone in bewilderment.

Yes, why indeed! thought Margarita reproachfully.

Several days later Jose and Margarita talked seriously about setting a wedding date. "Surely we will be better off in our own home," she said.

"Yes, I believe we are both ready for marriage," Jose replied with a nod. "We attend the same church; we know how to sacrifice; we are well-acquainted with hard work and responsibility." He paused meaningfully. "What would you think of one month from Christmas day?"

Margarita's face was radiant. "I think it would be the happiest day of my life."

"But I will wait as long as possible before asking your father for your hand," he added quietly.

One week before the proposed wedding date, Jose Maria asked his son, "When are you going to get married, Chemita?"

Jose stammered, "Next week, Papa. On Monday."

His father scowled and muttered something unintelligible under his breath. "I was afraid of that," he said. "You know how much we depend on your income."

"I know, Papa. But you receive an allotment from the government agencies because of your hand."

"Not enough," returned Jose Maria sharply. "And tell me, Chemita, how do you plan to support a wife?"

"I will manage somehow," said Jose stubbornly.

"But you are too young. You cannot marry without my permission."

"Then I ask your permission, Papa. I have made up my mind. Margarita and I want to be married next week."

For several moments his father appeared deep in thought. Finally he adjusted his shoulders and cleared his throat. "Very well, Chemita. Then we must do what is proper. We will go together to ask Sr. Peralta for his daughter's hand."

"I had hoped you would say that, Papa," sighed Jose in immense relief. The last thing he had wanted to do was to face Jesus Peralta alone!

At dusk the next day, Jose walked up to the door of Margarita's house accompanied by his father Jose Maria, his Uncle Marciano, and Brother Mercado. *There is safety in numbers,* he told himself. He knocked soundly, then turned to his father. "You go in, Papa. I will wait out here."

Magdalena greeted the three men and invited them inside while Jose, Jr. darted around to a side window to watch the proceedings. Jesus Peralta sat at a table drinking. Margarita stood across the room ironing.

After the men exchanged polite inquiries regarding one another's health, Jose Maria got right to the point. "We come representing my son Jose, to request your daughter's hand in marriage."

Jesus glanced with amusement toward the window. "Three of you representing one mere boy?" He looked at Margarita, who continued to iron, apparently oblivious of the weighty situation at hand. "Margarita, is this true what they say, that you plan to get married?"

Margarita did not look up. "Yes, Papa. It is true."

Jesus rubbed his chin thoughtfully. "I see," he said. "Very well. If you want to get married, you may." He stood up and, smiling generously, shook hands with each of his visitors. He was still smiling minutes later when the three men prepared to leave.

At the door, Jose Maria said to Margarita, "I want to see you in my house tomorrow. I want to speak to you . . . privately."

Margarita nodded. "Yes, of course," she said. "I will be there when I have finished my work in the lettuce field."

The men strode out then, and were joined by a delighted and much relieved Jose, Jr.

But once the door was shut, Jesus turned on Margarita, his face registering rage. "So you think you are smart, planning to marry and leave home!" He picked up a broom and began to strike her, chasing her around the room. She scrambled under a bed, but she couldn't escape the repeated "thwacks" of the broom handle against her flesh.

Later Jesus went out to get more whiskey. The younger children were asleep, and the house was quiet now except for one haunting sound—Magdalena sobbing. Margarita, still nursing her bruises, entered the kitchen and stared at her mother bent over the table, weeping.

"What is it, Mama? What's wrong?"

Magdalena struggled to compose herself. "Are—are you going to leave me?"

"Oh, Mama, what do you want me to do?" Margarita

reached out and squeezed her mother's shoulder. "I need a home, Mama. I've been roaming for so long. I've never really felt wanted. And you know Papa will not change."

"Oh, but he will change," said Magdalena urgently. "You must be patient with him."

Margarita gazed intently at her mother. "Mama, whatever happens, I'm going to get married."

That night Margarita tossed and turned, unable to sleep. She felt an ache inside that nothing could dispel—a pain provoked not by her father's vicious blows, but by the sight of her mother's tears.

When she finished work the next day, Margarita kept her appointment with her prospective father-in-law. With reserved politeness, Jose Maria showed her into the house. Apparently no one else was there.

"Come with me," he said, leading her into a dingy, cramped room. "You see this? This hovel is where my son Jose lives—your future husband!" He pointed to a bed with a dirty mattress and torn sheets. "You see this bed? This is where he sleeps. It is a miracle the blankets do not choke him." He gazed at her, his eyes narrowing. "My son has no money, no education, nothing at all to give you. Why do you want to marry him?"

Margarita met his gaze without flinching. "Because I love him," she said.

Their eyes remained locked for a long moment before Jose Maria broke away. "Very well, you know my son's circumstances," he said brusquely. "If you still insist on marrying him, don't you ever come crying to me for help. I have none to give."

"Do not worry," she told him firmly. "Chemita and I will never come begging to you."

As she turned to go, he called after her, "I tell you this, young lady, do not make a fool of my son!"

Without a reply she went out quickly and shut the door behind her.

Returning home that evening, Margarita reflected soberly on her future father-in-law's warning. He had obviously hoped to discourage her, to frighten her out of marrying his son. But his words had had the opposite effect. Margarita was more determined than ever that she and Jose would make it on their own. No matter how desperate the circumstances, never would they turn to either family for help. And true to their resolves, they never did.

Both Margarita and Jose discovered that there was much to do during the week before their wedding. Between them they had saved twenty dollars. They paid five dollars for the first month's rent on a tiny house two blocks from Jose's family and one block from the church. They put a down payment of $2.50 on some furniture—a bed, a dresser, and a kitchen table with two chairs. They would need $2.50 for the marriage license and ceremony, and another dollar for a week's supply of food. By the end of the week they had $2.50 left.

On January 25, 1937, the Hernandez and Peralta families met at the home of Brother Mercado for the wedding ceremony. Two of the church's deacons served as witnesses. Margarita was married in a borrowed dress; Jose wore an inexpensive suit and cowboy boots. But Margarita considered it a beautiful wedding. She felt incredibly happy and secure; she couldn't bear to let go of her husband's arm.

After the ceremony, around two P.M., Jose Maria suggested that everyone come to his house for a celebration dinner. After all, his house was close by, while the Peralta home was in Glendale, nine miles away. Besides, he figured Jesus Peralta looked a bit too tipsy for entertaining company.

As the wedding party headed for the Hernandez house, a little duplex on 11th Street, Sabina anxiously asked her husband, "What will we feed all these people?"

Jose Maria smiled reassuringly. "I'm sure you'll find something suitable."

One deacon brought a little cake, and Sabina made hot chocolate and coffee. "We are going to have eggs, *tortillas* and beans," she told her guests brightly.

"Eggs?" questioned Jose Maria.

"Yes, *eggs!*" she repeated, adding in a whisper, "It's all we have."

As Sabina cracked an egg into the frying pan, she emitted an exclamation of surprise. "Look, a double yoke."

"Ah, that means good luck," said the deacon.

Sabina cracked another egg and—amazing!—another double yoke. Everyone laughed. Another egg went into the pan, then another and another. Every egg had double yokes. The guests marveled over such an unusual occurrence.

"Surely you are going to be blessed," Brother Mercado told Jose and Margarita.

The families sat down together and ate heartily. They all agreed: the newlyweds would indeed be blessed.

About five P.M., as the guests prepared to leave, Jose Maria said loudly, "Wait, everyone, wait! We are going to pray." He instructed Jose and Margarita to kneel in the middle of the room. Then he and Sabina and Magdalena and Jesus formed a circle around the couple. Jose Maria placed Jesus' hands on the top of Jose, Jr.'s head and he put his own hands on Margarita's head. Then, in a strong, resonant voice he entreated God to bless his son and his son's new wife and the Christian home they were creating.

Since there was no money for a honeymoon, Jose and Margarita spent their wedding night in their little rented house. Both were painfully reserved. Margarita felt nervous, jumpy; she fought a sense of overwhelming anxiety.

Finally Jose said, "Well, we'd better go to bed."

"Okay," she replied reluctantly.

He climbed in on one side, she on the other. She curled up on the edge of the bed and turned her face to the wall. After an interminable silence, Jose said, "What's wrong, Margarita?"

She turned slightly. "I don't know, Chemita. I—I guess I'm afraid my father will show up. I'm afraid something will happen. I've run from him for so many years. What if he comes and spoils things now, just when we have a chance to be happy? I can't stop feeling afraid."

Gently Jose took her in his arms. "You must settle down, *mi amor*," he told her. "I know all you've gone through, but you must understand that you belong to me now. You are mine, and I am going to protect you. You don't have to be afraid anymore."

By the early hours of the morning Margarita felt secure enough, calm enough, to sleep.

At dawn she and Jose rose and went, as usual, to the field to work. That was the extent of their honeymoon.

ELEVEN

One morning about three months after her wedding, Margarita paid her mother-in-law a visit. The two women sat chatting amiably when suddenly Margarita jumped up and ran to the bathroom. Minutes later she returned, her face ashen.

"What's wrong?" asked Sabina.

"I don't know," said Margarita weakly. "Something's wrong with my stomach. For days now I haven't been able to keep anything down."

Sabina gave her a knowing smile. "Ah, you're pregnant already!"

Margarita's eyes grew wide. "Me? Pregnant?"

"Yes, you're going to have a baby."

With wonderment Margarita ran her fingertips over her abdomen. "I cannot believe it," she murmured. "I thought only very special women had children."

"Special?" scoffed Sabina in amusement. "Am I so special? I have had a dozen children!"

"What should I do?" asked Margarita. "How should I prepare myself?"

"Rest, eat well, see a doctor. He will tell you what to do."

That evening when she shared the news with her husband, Margarita was nearly ecstatic. "Imagine, me—having a baby!"

"A baby," Jose marveled over and over.

"Yes, Chemita," she said, hugging him, "our own little one."

Margarita spent a great deal of time the next week thinking about the birth of her child. There were many things she did not know, things she had never found the courage to ask her mother. No one dared talk openly about the secrets of marriage and childbirth, so a girl stumbled upon the secrets only as she married and bore children herself.

As a youngster, Margarita had supposed that babies were brought in the doctor's black bag. It had seemed perfectly logical. Her mother would become ill; the doctor would be summoned; he would stride into the room carrying his little black valise. A little while after he had shut the door, she would hear a baby's cry. Where else could the baby have come from if not from the doctor's mysterious black bag?

Now, of course, Margarita knew better. She knew the baby came from its mother's stomach. But one thing still puzzled her. How did the baby get out?

Finally the answer came to her. Surely God had supplied the navel for some worthwhile purpose. That had to be where the baby would come out. So in the days that followed, she began a faithful routine of cleaning and massaging her navel with olive oil.

A week later she paid another visit to her mother-in-law.

"How are you feeling?" asked Sabina, leading Margarita inside.

"Not too good. I still get sick a lot."

"Well, are you taking care of yourself?"

"Oh, yes," said Margarita. "I have been putting lots of olive oil on my navel."

Sabina's eyebrows raised and her mouth dropped open. "What? What are you doing?"

Hesitantly Margarita repeated herself.

Sabina extended her hand in a perturbed, coaxing gesture. "Tell me, who told you to take care of your navel?"

Margarita grew increasingly flustered. "I—I . . . isn't the baby going to come from there?"

"No!" cried Sabina. "Don't you know—?"

"No," replied Margarita in a small, meek voice, "I don't know."

Sabina jumped up, exploding with scorn. "Never have I seen a woman so stupid as you!"

"But—" Margarita was nearly in tears.

Emitting an exasperated sigh, Sabina leaned close to her daughter-in-law and whispered, "The way the baby was made, that's where it's going to come out."

Margarita's eyes registered incredulity, then stark comprehension. She stared quickly at the floor, a mixture of embarrassment and shame coloring her face.

Sabina patted Margarita's arm and said reassuringly, "It's all right. I have a surprise for you. I am going to have a baby too. Perhaps they will be born at the same time." She reached over and tilted Margarita's chin. "Come now, why such a long face?"

"It is nothing," replied Margarita uncertainly. "I am only wondering what to tell Chemita. He too thinks the baby will come from the navel!"

Once it had been established *how* their child would enter the world, Margarita and Jose were ready to tackle weightier matters. For example, their child's education.

"We must see to it that our baby has culture," Margarita told Jose one morning as she shaved him (a routine they had established from the beginning of their marriage).

"Yes, culture is very important," he agreed.

"Our David must be an educated man."

"David?"

"Yes, our baby's name will be David," said Margarita, carefully guiding the razor over Jose's chin.

"I did not know we had decided on a name."

"Yes. Long ago I prayed and told God if ever he gave me a child, I would name him David—after King David in the Bible."

"Hmm. David Hernandez. A good name," agreed Jose.

"I want to buy our David a piano," announced Margarita unexpectedly.

Jose flinched, his jaw just missing the razor's edge. He

glanced at the slight swelling of his wife's abdomen. "Our David is not yet ready to play the piano," he said matter-of-factly.

"But we should have it ready for him," argued Margarita. "You received a raise in pay from eight cents to ten cents an hour. We could pay two dollars a month for the piano."

Jose nodded. "Yes, *querida*, you have a good idea. Our son may be a great musician. We must give him that chance."

The next day Margarita purchased a Pianola, a player piano for the son that was not yet born. Neither she nor Jose could foresee that in this case the best of intentions would prove utterly fruitless. The piano would sit untouched for six years, and by the time young David would be ready for lessons, the beloved Pianola would be irreparably infested with rats.

The piano was, however, the only extravagance Jose and Margarita allowed themselves. Otherwise, their existence remained austere. In fact, to save money they built their baby's crib out of old tomato crates and painted only the side that showed.

Margarita was plagued with nausea throughout her pregnancy. She found that the only way she could keep water in her stomach was by eating lettuce. Only once did she experience an unbearable craving—and that for the most unlikely of foods at the most inopportune of times. It was the beginning of October and she was eight months pregnant when it struck her suddenly that she had to have watermelon. She awakened Jose in the middle of the night and said, "Chemita, I smell watermelon . . . I taste watermelon . . . I need watermelon!"

He turned over and mumbled sleepily, "There's no watermelon anywhere this time of year."

"Please, Chemita," she pleaded. "I must have watermelon. Feel how hard the baby kicks. He wants watermelon too."

"Very well," sighed Jose. "I cannot refuse both of you."

He got up, dressed in silence, and went out bravely into the streets of Phoenix on his curious mission. He arrived back home around three A.M. and handed Margarita a slice of melon he had found in an all-night restaurant. "Here's your watermelon, and believe me, it's the only slice in all of Phoenix!"

Greedily Margarita devoured the sweet, luscious melon. Immediately the baby stopped kicking, and minutes later Margarita was asleep. Only Jose lay awake, too invigorated by his long pilgrimage in the night air to sleep.

One morning four weeks later, shortly after Jose had left to take laborers to the cotton fields, Margarita trudged heavily to her mother-in-law's house. Sabina opened the door, holding her month-old baby Eloisa in her arms. "What's wrong?" she asked when she saw the expression on Margarita's face.

"I don't know," winced Margarita, holding her stomach. "Something's wrong. It hurts me."

Sabina pulled her inside. "You're going to have the baby now. You'd better get ready."

"The baby . . . now . . . today?" Margarita returned home slowly and awkwardly. She carried a big cast-iron tub outside, emptied countless buckets of water into it, heated the water, then dragged the heavy tub back inside the house. She bathed and dressed, then returned to Sabina's house around four P.M..

"How do you feel?" asked the older woman.

"The pains are getting very bad," replied Margarita.

An expression of anger settled on Sabina's face. "Where is that husband of yours? He should be here by now." She went and looked out the door. "Tell me, where are our men when we need them!"

Sabina strode to the kitchen and returned moments later with a bowl of homemade chicken soup. "You'd better eat this," she said. "You've got to have lots of strength."

Obediently Margarita swallowed the soup.

At six P.M. Jose's truck rumbled into the driveway. Sabina went to the door and shouted, "Get in here, Chemita!"

He jumped from the cab and sprinted toward the door. "What's wrong, Mama?"

"Get in here! Your wife is going to have the baby!" she exclaimed.

Jose brushed past his mother, went over and embraced his wife, and asked solicitously, "Do you have any fever, *mi amor?*"

"Fever?" echoed Sabina in disbelief. "What fever? She doesn't have any fever. She's going to have a baby. You go get her mother."

Jose hesitated, bewildered. "But it's nine miles to her mother's home in Glendale. Is there time?"

"Yes," said Sabina. "Go quickly. She needs her mother with her."

It was nearly ten-thirty before Jose arrived back with Magdalena. "I got here as fast as I could," he explained lamely to his seething mother. "Magdalena wasn't home, so I had to look for her all over the neighborhood."

At last they drove Margarita to a nearby maternity hospital where she remained in hard labor until eleven A.M. the next day, October 29, 1937. After long hours of struggling against severe contractions, Margarita had her boy. But he was disturbingly blue and he wasn't breathing. She watched the doctor spanking him over and over, but the infant wouldn't cry.

Margarita lay back exhausted, tense, desperate to hear some sound of life, anything. Those few moments seemed to last forever, but finally the blessed, beautiful cry came. Her baby was alive! Margarita's heart swelled with praises.

TWELVE

"Chemita, we have nothing to eat—no milk, no beans, no bread."

"I know, Margarita, but there is no money."

"Chemita, our David is nearly three, well beyond the age of nursing. He needs food." She patted the huge swell of her stomach. "And next month there will be another child to feed."

"How can I buy food when I am out of work?" lamented Jose. He paced the floor, shaking his head ponderously. "Times are very bad. Day after day I look for a job, but I have no training, no education. So who will hire me?"

"Well, we must eat," said Margarita, pulling on her shawl. "So I will pay your family a visit."

Jose looked up in surprise. "You will not ask my father for help—"

"Of course not," she said quickly. "Never would I do such a thing. I would die first. I will simply do . . . what I always do."

"Yes, I know your little scheme. I wonder if they know it too?"

"They have no idea," retorted Margarita. "Besides, I work hard for the little bit of food I bring home. And your father—with his disability and so many children, he receives plenty of food from the NRA and WPA."

"So do not stand there talking, Margarita. Go!" said Jose. "And perhaps today I will find a job."

With little David in tow, Margarita walked the short distance to her in-laws' house and was greeted at the door by her sisters-in-law Elena, Chuy, and Apolonia.

"Would you like some help today with the washing?" asked Margarita.

The girls laughed in delight. "You are so generous, Margarita," marveled Elena. "You know how we hate housework."

I hate it too, Margarita mused silently, but aloud she said, "I am glad to help you. Shall I gather wood to heat the water?"

"We have mountains of dirty clothes," said Chuy, "and our knuckles grow red from scrubbing."

"Then I will help you scrub," said Margarita lightly.

"Will you also make us your special tortillas by hand?" asked Apolonia. "No one makes them like you."

"I would love to make them," said Margarita, beaming.

Late in the afternoon, after the wash had been completed and dinner was on the table, Margarita said, "Well, now I must go home."

"Oh, no, don't go," said Elena. "You have worked so hard. Please, stay and eat with us."

"Very well, I will stay. But not for long. I must get home and cook dinner for Chemita," said Margarita. Silently she thought, *Ha! Cook what? There is not a crumb of food in the house!*

"Why don't you take him a burrito?" suggested Chuy.

"Yes, I suppose I could do that," replied Margarita casually.

That evening she burst in the door, exclaiming, "Chemita, look at the burrito I have for you! I tell you, I stuffed that tortilla so full—!" She stopped abruptly and stared at her husband. "What is it, Chemita? You—you look like you have been crying."

He came and took her in his arms, weeping. "I . . . I still can find no work."

Margarita began to cry too. "Tomorrow, my Chemita. Tomorrow!"

Over the next few days Jose returned home each evening with despair etched in his face.

"Still nothing," he said flatly when he came home the third evening. He looked down at his young son. "Why is David crying?"

"He has cried all day," sighed Margarita. "He does not like having only water to drink."

"He is so hungry," said Jose. "Look, his lips are white and dry." He scooped David up and bounced him in his arms to quiet him, then gazed at Margarita with sorrowful eyes. "We have not eaten in two days. What will become of us?" Tenderly he pressed David's head against his shoulder. "We are desperate, Margarita," he said quietly. "We must do something, or we will die."

The next morning, with fresh determination in his voice, Jose told his wife, "I have been thinking, Margarita. We are going to see the governor."

"What governor?" she asked.

"The governor of Arizona, Robert Taylor Jones. You know him, don't you?"

"No, not personally."

"But I remember before we were married, you worked for his campaign during the election."

"There were many of us working for him," explained Margarita. "I knew who he was, but I never talked to him."

"Well, today you will meet him, so go get ready." He reached for her hand. "Wait. First we will pray." Together they knelt beside the little kitchen stove and prayed, committing themselves afresh to God. Then they set out for the Capitol Building in downtown Phoenix.

Arriving at the Capitol, they climbed several flights of stairs to the governor's office on the top floor. Margarita, her body swollen with her second child, lumbered breathlessly. Each step was a challenge. Jose carried David who, fretful from hunger and dehydration, squirmed restlessly in his father's arms.

They were met by a guard in front of Governor Jones' office. "Where do you think you're going?" he demanded.

In broken English, Jose explained, "Me and my wife . . . we wish to see the governor."

"Do you have an appointment?"

"No, señor."

"You cannot see the governor without an appointment," said the man.

Margarita looked in dismay at her husband. "What should we do?"

Jose's expression hardened slightly. "Let's go back down," he said.

They made the long trek back downstairs to the street and sat down wearily on a Capitol grounds park bench.

"What now?" asked Margarita.

"It is almost noon," said Jose. "The governor has got to eat, so we are going to stay here until he comes down."

For the next half hour they kept a patient vigil and as Jose predicted, at the stroke of twelve the governor's entourage came down the steps and headed for his automobile. Jose spotted the governor—a tall, blond, well-built man with glasses. He had four guards with him—two beside him and two following behind.

As Jose stood up and confronted the official party, two guards stepped protectively in front of the governor.

"What do you want?" asked one, his tone clipped.

"I—I want to speak to Governor Jones," said Jose.

Margarita stepped forward beside her husband, awkwardly balancing David on one rounded hip.

The guard spoke confidentially to the governor, then turned back to Jose. "All right, mister. He says he'll talk to you."

Jose met the governor's curious gaze and struggled nervously to recall the appropriate English phrases. "Sir, I come not asking for you to give me anything," he said, his voice tremulous. "What I'm asking is for you to help me find work. I got my boy who has not eaten in two days. And my wife . . . as you see, she is pregnant. I have no job and I have no money."

With a sympathetic smile Governor Jones reached into his pocket, took out a ten-dollar bill, and handed it to Jose. "Young man," he said, "you take this money and go buy food for your family. Then return here tomorrow morning.

You can work as a gardener on the Capitol grounds for a few months until you get on your feet."

With that, the chief of state proceeded on his way.

For an instant, Jose stood dumbfounded, speechless. Then, finding his voice, he called after the man, "*Muchas gracias*, señor! How can I repay you?"

As the governor stepped into his car, he looked back momentarily and smiled at Jose, lifting his hand in a half-salute. A minute later, his automobile pulled away from the curb.

Jose whirled around to face Margarita and gleefully wrapped her in his arms. "God has answered our prayer!" he exclaimed, loudly enough for the passersby to hear.

The couple laughed—nearly sang—all the way home.

"Never will I forget the kindness of that wonderful man, our Governor Jones," vowed Margarita. "I have not known a more generous, compassionate fellow—besides you, my Chemita. I tell you this, our children and our children's children will know of his good deed to us at this time when we are most needy."

That day was a turning point for Margarita and Jose. For nearly three months he worked as a gardener on the Capitol grounds, saving his money for a truck so that eventually he could go into business for himself. On June 1, 1940, Margarita gave birth to a healthy little daughter, Delia, or Dee as she came to be called.

That summer, paying cash, Jose purchased first one small truck and then a second larger one for transporting workers to the cotton fields. A routine was quickly established. At four every morning, Jose and Margarita drove the trucks into the *barrios* to pick up workers. Often with their sleeping children strapped on their backs, the couple labored long hours picking cotton and selling watermelons to the other field hands. Their days were exhausting, but at least they had work—and an opportunity to be independent.

Jose purchased a parcel of land for two hundred dollars, bought a tiny two-room house for fifty dollars, and had it moved to the lot for one hundred dollars. In time he built a larger, brick home next door and converted the first house into a store called *"El Limoncito,"* or "Little Lemon." For a while Margarita managed the store. She sold a variety of groceries, candies, and soft drinks, as well as ice cream from a little soda fountain. Eventually the store became a refreshment center for the surrounding ghetto community.

Jose also developed a profitable brick and wood business. He drove out regularly to the desert and chopped dead, dry mesquite trees into logs and hauled them home to sell. Since most people had wood-burning stoves, the lumber sold well.

Adobe, an inexpensive material for constructing homes, was also very popular in the Phoenix area. Jose spent long hours in his adobe brick facility, combining mud with straw and various oils, supervising the men who waded around in the mud to mix it (there were no machines), and then pouring the mixture into molds or frames to dry. The dried adobes were removed from the frames by hand, stacked, then transferred by truck to the construction sites.

On October 1, 1941, Margarita bore her third child, another daughter, Norma. In every way life appeared on the upswing for the growing Hernandez family. They had their health, a comfortable home, a profitable business (several in fact!), and financial security. As Jose and Margarita had vowed, they were indeed making it on their own.

THIRTEEN

World War II was raging now, and people everywhere were going to the factories to help in the war effort. After hiring two men to drive their trucks to transport workers to the field, Jose and Margarita began working five days a week for Goodyear Aircraft. At night they attended the Goodyear training school. Margarita worked as a riveter, repairing damaged planes or crawling inside the wings to work on the electrical wiring. Jose was a rigger on the big machines that moved the wings from one area to another inside the gargantuan hangar.

During the days, Margarita and Jose left their two girls with Margarita's mother Magdalena, and David with Jose Maria and Sabina. The youngsters enjoyed staying with their grandparents. Young David especially liked walking to school each day with his Aunt Eloisa, just a month older than he. But even though circumstances were improving for his parents, David's life was far from problem-free. He was waging his own private war against fear—an overwhelming, irrational dread of death. It was a monumental burden for a six-year-old to carry.

The seed of fear had been planted unsuspectingly one Sunday night when David was only five. The family was still living in the little house they had purchased for fifty dollars, since the larger brick house was not yet completed.

Because of the war, tires were expensive and scarce, so the huge spare tire for the truck was kept in the living room (which served also as the only bedroom).

That night the family had just returned from church. Margarita sent David to the kitchen to get Dee's milk bottle, actually a Coca-Cola bottle with a nipple on top. The light was out in the living room. As David rushed in, he tripped on the tire. The pop bottle struck the metal rim and shattered. David screamed as a jagged piece of glass pierced his arm, severing a major artery. The wound began bleeding profusely.

Jose snapped on the light, yanked out his handkerchief, and quickly made a tourniquet on his son's arm. He picked David up and carried him out to the car as Margarita ran out with the girls and lifted them into the back seat. Jose drove at top speed down Washington Boulevard, blowing his horn and waving his hat out the window at intersections to ward off other drivers. He ran every stoplight and arrived in record time at the hospital emergency room six miles away, where David was promptly treated.

But the child's emotional wound could not be so easily healed. David had been stunned by the accident, his sudden, overwhelming weakness, and the terrifying gush of blood. He was convinced he was dying. *Death*—what was it like? It was an ugly, ominous word. No one had ever talked to him about death.

For many nights following the accident, David suffered harrowing nightmares, some so intense they caused him to fall out of bed. He dreamed over and over that he was plummeting from an airplane or falling from a tall tree, always severely injuring himself.

The fears might have faded in time had not David faced another crisis the following year. At the age of six he entered the hospital to have his tonsils removed, and the old anxieties surfaced again. He was once more facing the unknown . . . perhaps even death. To him they were one and the same.

As David was wheeled into the operating room, he screamed and thrashed hysterically. Orderlies held him down while two nurses strapped him to the table. A paralyzing terror gripped him as he felt the straps tightening around his ankles, his thighs, and his waist and arms. Then when he was powerless to move, when the agony of fear was about to explode inside him, someone clamped a thick black rubber mask over his face. There was the steady *drip . . . drip* of ether. As the hideous smell began to overpower his senses, David thought he would suffocate. Dazedly he wondered, *Is this what it's like to die?*

The next morning nurses brought David several flavors of ice cream to soothe his sore throat. But nothing was offered to soothe his fears.

David tried to push the recurring anxieties away. Finally he buried them in a crevice of his mind. But often they sprang unbidden into his consciousness. There was the time David and his Aunt Eloisa crossed the vacant lot on their way home from school. A heavy-set black man with a wooden leg lived nearby. As David and Eloisa crossed the lot, they spotted the man lying under an old car, repairing it. David was convinced the man was aiming a rifle straight at them. He and Eloisa exchanged panic-stricken glances. "Let's run!" she cried. They sprinted the final block home, positive that at any moment they would be shot. (In retrospect, David imagines that the poor old black man must have wondered what had gotten into those kids, running like scared rabbits.)

Another incident—infinitely more serious and tragic—left its imprint on David's impressionable, young mind. One day as he was playing in the front yard of his Grandmother Sabina's house, he spotted an airplane overhead. He watched perplexed. The plane was coming down, but there was no landing strip around. The aircraft dipped in the sky just two blocks away, disappearing over the rooftops. Immediately there was an earth-jarring explosion. Flames and black smoke billowed on the horizon.

For an instant David stood paralyzed. Then he ran toward the house just as his family rushed outside. The entire community gathered at the scene of the wreckage to survey the devastation. David winced at the sight of the sprawling debris, the charred earth, the dozens of scattered, broken bodies. Shock numbed him; he could not comprehend such sudden, senseless destruction.

That evening David pressed close to his mother's side, seeking comfort and reassurance. Margarita put her arm protectively around him and said, "You know, son, we feel so helpless when we see people hurt and dying . . . like those poor people in that plane crash. But there is a way you could help people who are hurt." She tilted his chin and looked him in the eye. "You could become a doctor, David. You would make a good doctor."

A doctor? It was a novel thought. The seven-year-old had been so plagued by his fears of death, it hadn't occurred to him that he could actually fight that mysterious, unpredictable enemy. But a doctor? The very idea was incomprehensible to a Mexican ghetto youngster who spoke little English and possessed only the most rudimentary knowledge of what the rest of the world was like.

While David struggled to cope with his recurring fears and marveled over the incredible possibility of someday becoming a physician, his parents continued to work dauntlessly to lift the family from ghetto status. Jose and Margarita leased forty acres of land on which they planted potatoes and watermelon. They hired laborers and brought in Jose's father, Jose Maria, to supervise the workers. They raised an impressive crop. Every week they filled a railroad boxcar with watermelons to be taken to San Francisco. The government bought everything they could grow.

Eventually Margarita's parents, Jesus and Magdalena, moved from Glendale to a house a couple of blocks from their daughter. Jesus still drank obsessively and had to be bailed out of the drunk tank with distressing regularity. It became almost a tradition for Margarita to go by the jail to secure her father's release, before taking the family to Sunday school and church. Jesus was a tremendous nuisance; no one in the family could manage him.

Except Margarita. Amazingly, she was the only one to whom he would listen, the only person he obeyed. Magdalena had finally washed her hands of her husband, reconciling herself to the fact that, indeed, he would never change. She focused all her love and attention now on Ralph, her youngest child and the only one remaining at home. All the other children were married, out on their own, and they wanted nothing to do with a drunken father who had so cruelly mistreated their mother.

Thus, the most improbable of events occurred. Margarita took her father into her own home to care for him and watch over him. She put him in charge of running "El Limoncito," and he managed the store surprisingly well. Apparently he had found his niche, for rarely now did he need to be rescued from the drunk tank.

While the war years may have thrown the rest of the world into turmoil, for Margarita and Jose life had assumed a blessed measure of stability, security, even predictability. Hard work and sheer determination had paid off. The grim days of poverty seemed far behind.

Then came 1945 and the end of the war. Both Margarita and Jose were laid off from the Goodyear plant. To supplement their income, they spent a season harvesting the fruit crop in California.

Shortly after their return to Phoenix, their daughter Dee developed a severe rash over much of her body. Medical expenses mounted as the couple consulted one doctor after another. The six-year-old was given multiple allergy tests, including fifty skin tests on her back in one day. A doctor in Nogales gave her calcium injections and suggested her parents take her to the coast to escape the heat. But no physician could accurately diagnose Dee's ailment. No medication brought relief. The bizarre disorder caused Dee's skin to peel in sheets, leaving her flesh bleeding and oozing. She lost the skin on her face five times.

For a year Dee suffered. Margarita never heard her daughter cry, but often she glimpsed the child in her room kneeling and praying. Every Thursday night the church people met in the Hernandez home to entreat God for Dee's recovery. Often the family gathered around an old Spanish Bible and wept over Dee's plight.

The illness also took a devastating toll on the family's finances. Jose was forced to mortgage their home to pay the fees of the numerous specialists; the brick and lumber business foundered as monetary resources were rapidly depleted.

In the summer of 1946, the Hernandez family journeyed again to California to harvest the crops. They had little money and were forced to sleep on the side of the highway. When they arrived in the San Jose area, they stopped beside the ocean and knelt on the beach to pray. Aloud, Margarita said, "Lord, what are you telling us? Here we are. We don't have any money. We don't have a place to go. We need your help. Our child Dee needs your help. We have cried so many times, seeing her suffer like this. Help us, Father, please."

After they had prayed, David and Norma dashed into the water to play. Dee lingered on the shore, watching wistfully.

"Come on in, Dee!" shouted David. "It's fun!"

Cautiously Dee splashed in after her brother. Margarita winced. What would the saltwater do to Dee's raw sores? But the child played happily, without a word of complaint.

The family camped on the beach that night; the next day the children again played in the ocean for hours. That evening Margarita noticed something unbelievable: Dee's skin was drying. The family knelt and prayed a second time, thanking God for his goodness. They stayed a few more days, and each morning the children scurried into the ocean to play. By the third day Dee's skin had cleared; no sign remained of the mysterious ailment. The family rejoiced, praising God for his miracle of healing.

In the fall the family returned to Phoenix, hoping to recoup some of their financial losses from the year before. Now if only their earnings from their harvesting venture in California would put new life into their faltering businesses at home!

In October Margarita became pregnant with her fourth child. When she was two months along, she began to hemorrhage and entered the hospital immediately. Over the next five months she bled frequently and had to be hospitalized each time. The doctors diagnosed her condition as "placenta previa," an abnormal—and potentially danger-ous—problem.

In May 1947, during her seventh month, Margarita suffered a massive hemorrhage and went into premature labor. Jose summoned her mother and a midwife who delivered the infant—a boy Margarita named Ronald. The child was tiny and extremely weak. Two days passed, and when the baby failed to improve, Jose brought in a doctor to examine his son.

"My little boy . . . Ronnie . . . how is he?" asked Margarita anxiously when the doctor approached her bedside.

The physician shook his head sadly. "I'm sorry, Mrs. Hernandez. This baby is not going to make it."

She stared wordlessly at the man. A searing memory sprang from the past—Margarita as a girl holding her baby brother Ramon, refusing to surrender him, as if by her very will she could propel life back into his still form. Now it was her very own son she was losing, her sweet little baby that God was asking her to surrender. She looked beseechingly at her husband. He took her hand and held it firmly.

A few hours later Ronald died.

The family held a simple graveside ceremony for the child. Before the coffin was lowered into the ground, Jose snapped a picture of David, Dee, and Norma in their Sunday clothes, standing stiffly, somberly behind their brother's open casket. The photo captured disarmingly the pathos of that moment—Jose's live children standing in the sunshine, keeping a mournful watch over the flower-wreathed death-cradle that held the child they would never know.

Stunned by the loss of their baby and facing certain bankruptcy as a result of Margarita's many hospitalizations, the couple took sober stock of their lives.

"All our savings are gone," said Jose. "The house is mortgaged, and the businesses have failed. We have nothing. We are back where we started when we were first married."

"What will we do?" asked Margarita.

"I think we should go to California. We can harvest the crops like we did before."

Margarita nodded. "That will be best for Dee too. She is still very weak, and I am afraid her illness will return if we stay here in Phoenix."

"Then let us prepare now to go," said Jose. "I am quite sure my parents would like to move into our house and take over the payments. This will make a good home for them."

Jose sold the better truck, keeping the dilapidated Ford for their trip. Shortly before they were scheduled to leave, Margarita approached her father and said, "We are moving to California, and I think you had better come with us. Get yourself ready."

"I don't want to go," said Jesus.

Margarita placed her hands on her hips and replied firmly, "I don't know where we are going to live, Papa. We could live under a tree. But you are going with us. If you stay here, you will just be a big nuisance. You will make my mother miserable . . . everybody miserable. You are safe only with me."

"What about your mama?" he asked. "Is she coming too?"

"No. Mama is staying here. She does not want to leave. Ralph has a good job now. He will support her."

Jesus grunted with disgust. "These days your mama thinks only of Ralph, no one else."

"And why not?" returned Margarita shortly. "You never gave her any love or attention. Now go pack your things. We leave tomorrow."

Her father's expression settled into a pout. "I don't want to leave my brass bed. It is the only bed I like."

Margarita thought a moment. "I tell you what," she said, "we are going to load your bed on the truck. We will fix it so you can sleep all the way to Los Angeles if you wish."

The next morning—a sunny June day in 1947—Margarita and Jose carried the brass bed outside and lifted it on to the truck. Then they packed the stove and the rest of their household items around and above it, leaving just enough space for her father to sleep. Obediently, an inebriated Jesus crawled into the bed, where he would sleep soundly for most of the trip.

The Hernandez family left for California with little more than faith in their pockets. They had only a few dollars for gas and food, plus a crate of watermelons and a crate of cantaloupes given to them by a friend who worked at the produce docks.

The family spent six tedious, uncomfortable days crossing the desert. Periodically they stopped along the road and gathered rocks to heat their *tortillas* and beans. Halfway across the scorching tundra, the truck's front wheels broke off and the truck sat down on its belly with a jolt. Jose spent nearly two days making repairs, and even when they pulled back on to the two-lane highway no one was certain the wheels would hold. When the weary travelers finally rumbled into Los Angeles, they hit a rut which sent their stove bouncing off the truck on to a busy street. Too mortified to go back and retrieve their possession from its spot in the center of traffic, Jose and Margarita drove on without looking back.

114

FOURTEEN

During the summer of 1947, the Hernandez family traveled to Wasco, California, near Bakersfield, for the potato harvesting season. Home became a makeshift tent pitched in the migrant camp beside the fields. After the harvest, the family moved north to the Santa Clara Valley where they secured contracts to harvest fields of tomatoes and sugar beets. They settled temporarily in an apricot orchard, where Jose built a lean-to shelter out of 3′ x 6′ fruit-drying trays. Their ceiling was the star-flecked sky above, and their beds were fruit boxes turned upside down (except for Jesus' brass bed, which remained outside). Jose went to the local county dump and found a large oil barrel which he filled half-full with dirt to fashion a mud stove. Margarita cooked outside, and tortillas and beans never tasted better! The Hernandez family labored together, working twelve-hour days, following the crops, picking potatoes, tomatoes, sugar beets, grapes, apricots, and plums.

The next year they rented a tiny house, formerly a chicken coop, on Felipe Avenue in San Jose. Margarita collected cardboard boxes from behind the local grocery stores and nailed them to the walls, then painted the cardboard with water colors to create her own special "wallpaper." In spite of the fact that the *San Jose Mercury News* labeled their street "the blighted area of San Jose," the

Hernandez family felt pleased to have a home of their own once more. They began to attend a little Mexican Baptist church in a nearby Mexican neighborhood called "*Sal Si Puedes*" ("Leave if you can").

Shortly after settling in San Jose, Margarita started working at a local cannery and Jose purchased a dump truck with which to haul salt from the Mt. Eden and Hayward areas to the Oakland shipyards. Eventually he owned two diesel trucks and made long-distance hauls from California to Oregon and Arizona, carrying hay, cement, fruit, or lumber. From 1947 through 1955 Jose drove his trucks for a living and was often away from home for days, even weeks at a time.

Jose faced several close calls while making his runs. Once, while going down the "grapevine" south of Bakersfield, his air brakes gave out. As the loaded truck gained momentum, Jose blinked his lights and sounded his horn until the driver in the next lane got his message. The man swung his truck over in front of Jose's and braked several times, allowing their bumpers to hit until Jose's rig slowed down enough for him to gain control.

Sometime later a similar experience produced near-tragic results. Once again Jose's brakes failed and his truck swiftly gathered speed. Snow was falling heavily, and the highway was icy. This time there were no other drivers to signal for help. In moments Jose's truck was totally out of control.

As Jose raced toward a curve, he decided to run the vehicle off the side of the road. The road curved to the left and the truck jackknifed to the right, careening off the highway over a treacherous gully. In that instant, Jose felt a power beyond his control pulling him over to the rider's side of the cab. He shoved open the door, jumped free, and tumbled onto the side of the highway. The truck shot over him, plunging over massive boulders and mountainous brush into a deep ravine fifty feet below. The vehicle was completely demolished, but Jose suffered only minor cuts and bruises.

"An angel of God saved me," he later told his astounded family. "The force should have thrown me out the driver's side where I would have been crushed by the truck. But something pulled me out the rider's side so I fell clear. When

I looked up and saw the bottom of that monstrous rig and those back wheels sailing over my head, I knew I was part of a miracle.''

The Hernandez family praised God, vowing never to forget Jose's amazing deliverance from the runaway truck.

Occasionally Margarita and the children went along on Jose's overnight runs, so that she could take the wheel and drive while Jose slept. As David grew older, he alone sometimes accompanied his father on the runs, driving while Jose napped. David, short for his age and slight in build, learned to drive almost before his feet could reach the pedals. When he drove, he always remained watchful for the highway patrol, his eyes darting from one rearview mirror to the other, ready to wake his father and switch places at a moment's notice. Once, while driving down the Pacheco Pass into Los Banos, David's heart leaped as he spotted a patrol car approaching his truck. But he heaved a sigh of relief when the officer passed by without noticing young David at the wheel.

In 1950, when David was only twelve, his father bought him his first car, a '39 Chevy in perfect condition. The Chevy had fog lights, an immaculate paint job, a spotless running board, and bumpers that shined. David was delighted. Never had he dreamed of owning anything so beautiful.

"Son, this will be yours when you are of age,'' said Jose.

But David couldn't resist trying out his new automobile. One Sunday night he decided to drive the family to church. A heavy fog hung over the Santa Clara Valley. David traveled between twenty-five and thirty-five miles per hour, even though he couldn't see more than fifteen feet ahead. It occurred to him that he could see better if he stuck his head out the side window. So he rolled down the window and craned his neck outside.

Suddenly a parked car loomed up before him. By the time David pulled his head back inside and slammed on the brakes, he had struck the vehicle and knocked it thirty feet into a ditch. Horrified at what he had done, David scrambled out of the car and ran to the other vehicle. He found a badly shaken young woman and her little son. They were unhurt.

"Our car stalled,'' the woman told him weakly. "With the

fog so bad, we didn't know where we were. My husband went for help."

David and his father inspected the damage to the two automobiles. The woman's car was barely scratched, but David's cherished Chevy was nearly ruined. The wheels would turn only to the left. Somehow he managed to drive home, but right turns were nearly an impossibility, executed only by maneuvering the car backward and forward time and again.

David was heartsick, fighting back tears of anger and frustration. "I never want to touch a car again," he told his parents vehemently.

"You'll change your mind, son," his mother assured him.

"I think you've learned some important lessons tonight," observed Jose.

"Lessons!" protested David. He wasn't sure he wanted to hear what they were.

"Yes," said his father soberly. "You've discovered that even the best of things can be destroyed, and therefore must be handled carefully." He placed a reassuring hand on the boy's shoulder. "And, son, you've experienced one of the dangers of driving and have seen how easy it is to jeopardize the lives of other people. I think you're beginning to learn that almost everything in life involves an element of danger and risk."

For nearly a month David agonized over the accident. How close he had come to injuring—perhaps even killing—innocent people! And he had ruined his beautiful automobile! Would he ever love anything as much as he loved that car?

FIFTEEN

When Jose first moved his family to California in 1947, Margarita's father, Jesus Peralta—and his cherished brass bed—went with them. Jesus, with his history of alcoholism and abusiveness, had always been a threat and a bother to his family. He had rarely held a job. But shortly after his arrival in Mt. Eden, he was given a job on a ranch driving a Caterpillar tractor. He worked steadily, and in time became surprisingly self-sufficient. Even more amazing, he stopped drinking.

While Jesus remained basically a remote, private individual, he gradually became accustomed to life in his daughter's home—Margarita's good cooking, the family's habits of sharing and expressing concern for one another, and their unalterable routine of attending church twice every Sunday and on Wednesday nights.

At first Jesus merely tagged along to the Mexican Baptist Church for something to do. Then one day he dusted off his violin and took it with him. He met informally with several other musicians in the church. One played the accordion, another the trumpet. Margarita joined them on her guitar. The group practiced together frequently and began performing special numbers in church. The changes occurring in Jesus Peralta's life were not sudden, but they were no less dramatic. He was becoming a sober, rational, productive member of the Hernandez household.

But for some time Jesus clung to one habit that greatly distressed Margarita—smoking. The children, too, hated their grandfather's foul-smelling cigarettes. Nevertheless, one Christmas when David was in the fourth grade, he decided to give his Grandfather Jesus a carton of cigarettes. Margarita made the purchase at a nearby corner store adjoining a service station, and David wrapped the gift himself. On Christmas morning he handed the package to his grandfather and watched expectantly as the dour-faced man fumbled with the ribbon and tissue paper. For a long moment Jesus stared at the shiny new carton of cigarettes. Then he looked up at David, a rare expression of emotion on his face. "You would give me these even though you hate my smoking?" he asked in bafflement.

David smiled and shrugged. "Sure, why not, Grandpa? I wanted to please you."

That evening, without a word to his family, Jesus put away the unopened carton. For the rest of his life he never touched another cigarette.

In 1950 Jesus' wife, Magdalena, and her youngest son Ralph moved to California, into the house next door to Jose and Margarita. Although Jesus remained for some time in his daughter's home, he resumed a tenuous relationship with his wife.

In fact, for the first time in his life Jesus was ready to work at his marriage. He supported his wife, took her to church each Sunday, and in his own private way attempted to show Magdalena that he cared for her. But, sadly, Magdalena too had changed. Too many years of hurt and disappointment had turned her love for Jesus sour. It was as if she had vowed never again to allow herself to be vulnerable to her husband. What's more, she had learned that she could survive, even be happy, without him.

Still, eventually Jesus moved back permanently with Magdalena. She washed his clothes, prepared his meals, and cared for him when he was ill, but emotionally she remained detached. She was more interested now in her grandchildren. They received the love and attention which in earlier years she had given unconditionally to Jesus. So devoted did Magdalena become to her grandchildren that she often spoiled the youngsters, giving in to their whims, plying them with candy (she collected bottles along the roadside to earn money for their sweets), and defending them vociferously against parental chastisement. In fact, whenever Magdalena caught her daughter whipping one of the children, she would chase Margarita around the room with a broom, shouting, "You leave my grandchild alone!"

In 1955, an accident involving Magdalena paved the way for Jesus' conversion to Christ. One afternoon Margarita received a phone call from her father; he sounded frightened. "Your mama . . . my Magdalena . . . she has been run over by a car," he told her, his voice quavering. "She's hurt bad. Come quickly."

Margarita drove immediately to the intersection and found her mother still lying on the pavement. She knelt and comforted the stricken woman until the ambulance arrived. Magdalena suffered internal injuries and a broken arm and leg. She remained in the hospital for a month.

In the years following Magdalena's accident, Jesus continued to mellow. He became increasingly involved in the church. He took care of his wife uncomplainingly while she was ill. And he was quietly devoted and respectful to both Magdalena and Margarita. In 1960, he made a full commitment of his life to Christ.

Often Margarita told her mother, "Papa has changed. He is a wonderful man now. You should be nice to him. Can't you see how he is different?"

In bitter irony Magdalena—the woman who years before had been so certain her alcoholic husband would change—now merely shook her head and snapped, "No, I don't believe it. He has not changed."

In 1965, Magdalena died without knowing the closeness with her husband that he had hoped fervently to establish. She had loved the Lord, trusted him; but the emotional wounds inflicted by Jesus Peralta were so deep and extensive they never healed.

After Magdalena's death, Jesus moved back in with his daughter and remained in Margarita's home until his death in 1975. He sought Margarita's advice about everything—where to go, what to buy, whom to see. He refused to stay with his other children. Once Margarita took him to her sister's house for a visit. Two days later he caught a plane home. When Margarita's brother Ralph asked their father to come live with his family, Jesus replied, "No, I don't have any business over there."

Jesus' final years revolved around the Mexican Baptist Church in San Jose. He was always the first one at services, and whenever the church needed money Jesus dipped into his Social Security savings for a few dollars, or a hundred, or as much as 500 dollars. In 1969, when a new church was built on 9th Street, Jesus was at the site nearly every day, working unrelentingly beside his son-in-law Jose to construct the new edifice.

In September 1975, Jesus suffered a stroke and was hospitalized. Then he developed pneumonia. "There's nothing we can do," the doctor told Margarita. The family spent the night watching over Jesus, grieving over his suffering.

Long forgotten memories flickered in Margarita's mind. She recalled how as a child, before she knew the Lord, she had hated her father. Those days belonged to another lifetime. Margarita had taken care of Jesus for so long; he had become very important to her. It was a strange paradox. She was Magdalena's misbegotten child, the daughter he would not claim because he was not her father; he was the once brutal stepfather she had once wanted to kill. The most unlikely of beginnings, but over the years, through Christ, they had formed a unique bond. They had become different persons. They had learned to love as father and daughter.

That night, while Margarita sat faithfully by his bedside, Jesus slipped into a coma. He died at three P.M. the next day.

PART FOUR
DAVID HERNANDEZ

SIXTEEN

When it came to the development of her children, Margarita Hernandez put the emphasis on *study*. Her philosophy was, "Strength, time, and intellect are but lent treasures from God." She was determined to see that her children received the best possible education, and that they used their talents to honor the Lord.

From the time her youngsters were small, Margarita pondered ways of stretching their horizons, of pushing them beyond the constricting boundaries of ghetto life. Often she told Jose, "I want my children out of this ghetto. I want something better for them. Here we have nothing."

When David was only seven, Margarita telephoned the YMCA one day and asked, "Do you have special programs for children?"

"We have hobby classes in the afternoon," a man replied. "You know, where the kids make model airplanes and stuff."

"Well, I have a son," said Margarita in a confiding tone. "He doesn't know much English. We speak only Spanish at home."

"That's all right," said the man. "Bring him over."

That afternoon Margarita dropped her reluctant son off for the two-hour class. David, frightened and close to tears, felt painfully out of place. This was the first time he had stepped out of his own safe, predictable enviroment to be surrounded by Anglo-Saxon children. He wasn't sure he could even communicate with them. But before the class concluded, he was actually enjoying himself. The way Margarita saw it, she had helped her son to cross an important bridge into the world at large, a world that would someday become her son's.

Jose, too, was determined that his son learn basic lessons to help him cope with life and become a man of integrity and worth. Just as *education* was an important word to Margarita, so *responsibility* was a favorite in Jose's vocabulary. Whatever it took, he would make his son a responsible person. Lessons occurred spontaneously, whenever life and the daily mundane routine offered an opportunity.

One Saturday Jose was repairing the flatbed in his diesel truck, methodically drilling several bolt holes. He had to work with slow precision, for one wrong move could break the metal drill. Thirteen-year-old David watched intently.

Jose glanced at his son, then asked, "You want to try it?"

"I sure would," said David eagerly. He took over the job, worked confidently, then fumbled and broke the drill. He felt heartsick.

Jose gazed patiently at the boy. "Well, son," he said, "I've got six dollars in my pocket, and I got to have this flatbed fixed up for hauling on Monday. So let's go get another drill."

"But that money is all you have for food this week," protested David.

"We'll get by," said Jose, climbing into the cab. They drove to the store, purchased a new drill for two dollars, and returned home. David tried again—and broke the second one. Furious with himself, he looked up despairingly at his father.

Jose's expression remained placid. "Let's get in the truck again, son," he said matter-of-factly.

David could hardly keep from crying. "But you have only four dollars left for food—"

Jose shrugged. "Food we can always manage one way or another. But to teach you a lesson, sometimes it costs money. More than that, it costs you to realize what it takes to be patient and productive."

David remained silent. He would have felt better if his father had taken him over his knee and spanked the daylights out of him.

They drove to the store, spent another two dollars, and returned with the drill. David looked hesitantly at his father and mumbled, "Dad, I don't want to do it this time. You do it."

Jose placed a reassuring hand on the boy's shoulder. "Son, we know you have broken two of these, but by now you should have just the right touch."

Gingerly David tried again. He worked with agonizing concentration. At last he accomplished the task. He grinned proudly at his father. Jose was beaming too. David would never forget the lesson he had learned that day; nor would he forget his father's enduring patience and his unswerving confidence in his son's abilities.

Jose Hernandez also instilled a sense of responsibility in his son through his consistent discipline. Never did he punish in anger. Whenever David misbehaved, Jose would sit down with him and calmly state the particular misdeed and the number of "spanks" the boy would receive. Then he would add, "Son, I sure hate to spank you, but if I don't I will be betraying myself and my responsibility."

David would grit his teeth and wish that his dad would just keep quiet and give it to him.

But no matter how much David and his sisters dreaded their father's spankings, they feared their mother's even more. Margarita had no methodology for discipline—and no control. She reacted out of anger, grabbing a broom, a belt, or whatever was handy. Beatings spawned by outrage— Margarita had known no other form of discipline. She recognized that her bursts of anger were wrong, but the pattern of behavior was ingrained from childhood and difficult to break.

Still, when it came to administering punishment, Margarita and Jose found a solution to maintaining a united front before the children. They settled on a private signal between themselves. Whenever Margarita lashed out uncontrollably at one of the children, Jose made it a point not to interfere. Instead, he would say with deliberate nonchalance, "Go ahead, Margarita. Give him another one." What he really meant was, *You better quit right now!* Margarita would calm down and release the youngster, and the incident would be over. She had saved face; he had saved the children from possible harm. And no one was the wiser. David and his sisters did not discover their parents' "secret code" until they reached adulthood.

In 1950, when David began his final year of grade school, his parents started thinking seriously about where he would attend high school. Determined that her son be educated at a private boarding academy, Margarita began applying for scholarships. But she soon discovered her efforts were in vain. "Ah, they have nothing for a poor Mexican boy from the ghetto," she lamented to Jose. Nevertheless, with or without a scholarship, David was accepted for the next fall at Brown Military Academy in San Diego.

Six months later, in the spring of 1951, Jose and Margarita considered the possibility of moving back to Phoenix, tentatively planning to leave California when David entered Brown Academy. The idea grew more probable when Jose met a couple who had a house to sell in the Camelback area of Phoenix. Jose was interested, but neither he nor Margarita could take off time from work to travel to Phoenix to inspect the property.

Then Jose had an idea. He said to David, "Son, you are out of school for Easter vacation. Why don't you go take a look at the place and see what you think? The owners are driving to Phoenix for a couple of days anyway. Maybe you could go along."

Thirteen-year-old David looked thoughtful. "You mean you and Mom will go by what I say?"

"Yes," said Jose. "If you think we should take the house, we will. If not, we'll stay here. It will be up to you."

David nodded. It never occurred to him to question how he would make such a momentous decision regarding his family's future.

Early the next morning David left with the couple on the eighteen-hour drive to Phoenix. After arriving at the couple's home, David looked around the house and explored the property, taking pictures. He even collected soil samples in little jars. When he had finished his inspection, he asked the couple to drive him to town where he was to meet his Aunt Elena. After spending the night with his aunt's family, David rejoined the couple for the trip back to California.

At home, radiating self-confidence and pride in a job well done, David reported his findings to his waiting parents. He gave the Arizona property a negative verdict; he felt it wasn't worth the price. David's word was final. The Hernandez family remained in California.

As the fall of 1951 approached, Jose and Margarita turned their attention to preparations for David's attendance at Brown Military Academy. Jose arranged for David to meet with the dean of the academy at the St. Francis Hotel in San Francisco. One week before the appointment, the Hernandez family went for a "going away" drive and informal counseling session along the picturesque Santa Cruz coastline. As David gazed out the window, an intriguing sign caught his eye: MONTEREY BAY ACADE-MY.

"Is that a military school?" questioned David.

"I don't know," said Jose. "Let's find out."

Jose drove to the academy, located in Watsonville. The family looked around and even managed to meet briefly with the principal. They learned that the school was a Christain co-educational academy. When they drove away from the academy a couple of hours later, they all shared the same startling conviction: This was the school David should attend.

"But without a scholarship, how will we pay the tuition or buy school clothes?" asked David soberly.

"We will trust the Lord to provide," replied Margarita.

The following week David was enrolled at Monterey Bay Academy. Margarita provided her son with a "new" wardrobe from *La Gloria*, the Salvation Army secondhand store. A few days later, Jose and Margarita drove David to the academy for the fall semester. Only thirteen, David had never lived away from home and knew no one on campus, except the principal. As he stood watching his parents' old

'37 Chevy sedan disappear into the distance, he wondered where his earlier self-confidence had gone. He felt dismayingly alone, vulnerable. He couldn't help wondering what he had gotten himself into.

The next few weeks were a nightmare for David. His loneliness was nearly overwhelming. He was too homesick to eat. He walked in his sleep. He wept during his private moments of devotion. Every day he wrote two or three letters home. It was scant relief to learn that his parents were enduring the same heartache of separation and that on their way back to San Jose, not once but several times they had almost returned to take him home.

When at last David overcame his homesickness, he did exceptionally well at Monterey Bay Academy. He made friends, became involved in campus activities, and earned impressive grades. He proved he could step out on his own, overcome personal anxieties, and meet the rigorous demands and standards of the academic world.

That spring of 1952, David received a call from a professor at San Jose State, for whom he had picked apricots the preceding year. "David, I want to be a camp director in the Santa Cruz Mountains this summer," explained the man, "but that means being away from my ranch during harvest season. I'd like to know if you could help me out."

"Certainly," replied David. "What do you want me to do?"

"Everything," came the quick response. "Take full responsibility of the ranch. Hire the workers, harvest the apricots, transfer the fruit to the sulfur houses, have it cut and processed, and of course pay the laborers. Do you think you can handle it?"

"Yes, I don't foresee any problem," said David pluckily. He was all of fourteen years of age.

With optimistic aggressiveness, David tackled his summer position as overseer at the orchard, located on an extremely steep hillside east of San Jose. He hired nearly twenty people to pick and process the fruit, and he used the professor's two small Ford trucks for transporting the apricots from the orchard to the processing shed.

Everything proceeded smoothly—until the transmission

went out on one truck while David was driving a full load of fruit up the hill. Feeling responsible because of his own inexperience in driving, David summoned his Uncle Vincent to repair the vehicle. David paid for all the replacement parts.

Toward the end of summer, the same thing happened to the second truck. Again David paid the bill. By the time the crop had been harvested, the fruit processed and dried, and the money counted, David realized a zero profit for the entire summer. He felt devastated. He had poured all his strength and time into three months of grueling labor—and he had nothing to show for it. There was no money for clothes or fall tuition. Once again he would have to select his wardrobe from *La Gloria*.

"At least it was a valuable experience," Jose told his disappointed son.

"Some experience!" returned David glumly. "I learned how to break trucks and put them back together."

Jose put a reassuring arm around the boy. "Son, it's not the money that counts. It's the experience of learning how to handle people, how to manage money, how to get a job done right. You can't put a price tag on experience like that."

Maybe not, mused David silently. But in this case, he wouldn't have minded a little less experience and a little more cash!

SEVENTEEN

One day during his sophomore year at Monterey Bay Academy, David and a half-dozen of his classmates decided to take a walk down by the beach abutting the school property. As they reached the opening of the storm drain, which spanned an eighth of a mile from the campus to the beach, one of his friends boldly crawled inside. Impulsively, a second boy followed, then a third.

David, valuing peer approval above almost anything else, accepted the challenge and crept in on his hands and knees too. With scarcely a moment's hesitation, the remaining youths squirmed into the narrow tunnel after him.

For the first fifty feet the shaft was filled with the echoing sounds of their laughter and chatter. But shortly the passageway grew black as tar. Their voices ceased quickly. David couldn't see a thing; he couldn't stand, turn around, or back up. He could hear only the hollow thumping noises of the boys ahead and behind him. He suspected that like himself, they were having second thoughts about what they had gotten themselves into.

For David, it was more than second thoughts. Panic clutched him—the horror of absolute darkness, a throbbing claustrophobic anxiety, and worst of all the disquieting realization, *I could die in here!* As he wormed forward through mud, gravel and debris, long dormant fears of death sprang up and taunted him. Childhood terrors became grisly phantoms of doom, harassing, reminding him, *There's no turning back . . . no turning back. You've got to see this through . . . or die!*

David closed his eyes and prayed as he clambered on exhaustedly through his tight, musty prison. After a grimly interminable crawl, David caught a faint glimmer—yes, a speck of light in the distance. He could see the other side . . . the world of daylight and land and sky! His companions were moving more quickly now. He glimpsed the rays of light projecting sporadically over their eager, lumbering, uncoordinated torsos. The chatter began again . . . followed by shouts and laughter and finally loud hoorahs. The boys were home free!

The haggard, mud-drenched youngsters scrambled awkwardly out of the storm drain, gulping fresh air, gingerly trying sore muscles. Ignoring raw hands, torn trousers, and scrubby knees, they congratulated one another for displaying magnificent bravery. They were careful not to cast blame for a most foolish and dangerous escapade, nor would anyone admit that he had been the slightest bit afraid.

At Monterey Bay Academy, every student had to perform manual labor, for which he was paid fifty cents an hour. Students worked two to three hours a day in the cafeteria, the laundry, the dairy, or on the campus farm; they served as paper-graders, mechanics, clerks, even garbage men. During David's first year he worked in the poultry department, collecting, examining, and separating eggs. Such tasks reaffirmed what his parents had always taught him—that labor has dignity.

In David's sophomore year, he worked as a gardener for the head of the science department, a gifted, older, unmarried woman. She took a special academic interest in David, eventually hiring him as her lab assistant and encouraging him to pursue a career in science. During his last two years at MBA, David corrected biology, chemistry, and geometry papers; and through this professor's recommendation, he was granted the rare opportunity of teaching lab science to his fellow classmates.

Since David wasn't convinced which profession he wanted to pursue, he joined nearly every school organization, including the journalism, creative writing, and Spanish clubs, and the Future Teachers of America. At times he considered becoming a missionary teacher. His father often suggested that he enter the ministry. His mother, of course, never entertained the possibility of any career for her son except medicine.

In his eagerness to explore every educational and cultural opportunity at MBA, David also became thoroughly involved in the music program. He took trombone lessons, played the piano, formed a quartet, and joined the orchestra and choir.

David was on the honor roll every semester. Yet for some time, he struggled painfully with the English language. His vocabulary was weak; he was constantly forced to turn to the dictionary for the meaning of words. Gradually he became obsessed with the dictionary, vowing never to turn the page of a textbook until he understood every word he had read. He began making lists of words to add to his vocabulary, usually fifteen to twenty new words each day. He discovered that if he looked up a word, wrote it down, then tried it on three persons, that word became his own. Thus, a dictionary and a thesaurus became his constant companions.

While he applied himself diligently to a variety of intellectual pursuits in high school, David also learned a great deal about comradeship and physical competition. A favorite game on campus was "rough-house"—essentially basketball without any rules. Once a month, on a Thursday night after study period, the upperclassmen took on the lowerclassmen in the school gymnasium.

David, smaller in stature than many of his classmates, felt a real need to assert himself. Often he ended up at the bottom of the pile, with a dozen hefty bruisers sprawled on top of him. Still, he forged ahead, struggling to make baskets, enduring the sore muscles. If nothing else, he learned how to take a beating.

One of David's most hilarious experiences occurred one day after a huge mountain of manure had been delivered to fertilize the soil behind the boys' dorm. It rained hard that day, thoroughly soaking and softening that ten-foot mound. Several of the upperclassmen were struck that evening with what they considered a brilliant idea. They decided to "baptize" several of the underclassmen. They "recruited" a number of unwitting, unwilling candidates and dunked them into the sodden, malodorous heap. Word spread swiftly that the upperclassmen were ganging up on the lowerclassmen. Within minutes the entire dorm was emptied as the boys rushed to the defense of their comrades. One after another, heads were pushed down into the cold, reeking muck; the hapless victims burst up coughing, spitting and sputtering. Pandemonium reigned.

Hearing the commotion, the dean ran out and stared in horror at the turbulent free-for-all in the refuse. "Let's have some order here!" he shouted, but his words were lost in the noisy melee and the miasma of dung.

Eventually order was restored, and the youngsters lined up without argument before the one outside shower. But it would be several days before they could completely erase the stench that had settled ignominiously on the male student body of Monterey Bay Academy.

During David's final year at MBA, he took pre-entrance examinations for college and underwent extensive career counseling. Since his tests revealed that he was best qualified for some area of science, he decided to enter college as a pre-med student. Margarita was delighted, though unsurprised. For the next eight years she would uncomplainingly put every paycheck she received from her job at the Levi Strauss Company toward her son's education.

In the fall of 1955, David entered Pacific Union College in Angwin, California, and promptly fell in love. Surprisingly, Ramona wasn't a college girl, but a new convert in his own home church in San Jose. She was an attractive, intelligent Mexican girl, five years older than David.

At first his parents were disturbed over the relationship. They argued that Ramona was too old for him and came from a "worldly" background. Margarita even threw a temper tantrum—weeping, screaming, and stalking angrily around the block during one of David's weekend visits home.

In tears David told his dad, "Mom just won't give me a chance to think for myself. How can I return to college with her so upset?"

Jose simply put his arm around David and said, "Don't worry, son. She will come under control again. She always does."

Surprisingly, not only did Margarita learn to accept her son's new romance, but after a few months both she and Jose became very fond of Ramona. They even began to urge David to marry her.

But David was away at college and meeting other pretty young ladies who were available for companionship when Ramona, in San Jose, was not. Besides, David sensed that in some obscure way he and Ramona were competing with each other, that perhaps she needed to feel she was better than he. Her attitude raised an unspoken barrier between them, gradually dampening his feelings for her. Although he and Ramona corresponded frequently, letters were a poor substitute for dating. As his affection continued to wane, he wondered how to tell Ramona. He simply could not find the courage.

During David's second year of college, he became president of the Northern Baptist Mexican Young People's Convention, a group of sixteen churches. He became deeply involved in their programs and organized large get-togethers every couple of months. He continued to date Ramona whenever he was in San Jose. So obsessed had David's parents become with Ramona that they impulsively purchased an engagement ring for him to give her. David put it away, not ready or willing to comply with their wishes.

Through his junior and senior years of college, David felt the pressure increasing from his parents and Ramona for a serious commitment. "She will make you a perfect wife," Margarita told him time and again. "She is Mexican, she loves the Lord, and she is smart and mature. And look how much she loves you. You are her whole life!"

David felt dismayed. How could he ever tell Ramona it was time for them to go their separate ways? Not only would he be breaking her heart, but he would be disappointing his parents as well. So, as he had done in the past, he let the matter ride.

On October 28 of David's senior year, he began the competitive three-day pre-entrance examination for medical school. That same day Margarita Hernandez went into labor and delivered her fifth child, a daughter she named Dana. David learned of the birth two days later, after he had completed his tests. His father telephoned and said, "You have a baby sister. Do you want to come home?"

"Of course!" David hopped into his car and drove straight to San Jose. Since his own birthday was October 29, he was one day short of being twenty-one years older than his new little sister Dana.

In the spring of 1959, David received his B.A. degree in biological sciences from Pacific Union College. That fall he entered Loma Linda University School of Medicine. Because of the distance, the demands of medical school, and a distressing lack of funds, David's trips to San Jose grew more infrequent. No longer able to put off the inevitable, he wrote Ramona, explaining that there was no use pretending they had a future together.

Ramona was crushed; Margarita was furious. She telephoned her son, insisting, "You don't know what you are doing. You don't know what you're going to lose out on!" Even David's sister Dee was upset. In David's absence, Ramona had become a virtual member of the Hernandez family.

David and Ramona saw each other one last time when she briefly visited Southern California. They had dinner together, then she flew on to Hawaii to assume the leadership of a home for wayward girls. The evening confirmed what they both already knew—there was nothing left between them but friendship. Ramona was a fine girl, a wonderful person, but she and David simply weren't meant for each other.

In spite of his long hours of study and the strenuous schedule at medical school, David soon became romantically involved with Joyce, a local young lady, a Seventh-Day Adventist and dental hygienist. She was a beautiful Anglo girl and David was enchanted. They began dating steadily.

During David's sophomore year at Loma Linda, he traveled to San Francisco to apply for a loan from the Bay City Baptist Union. His mother's faithful paychecks and his own summer earnings barely covered the 3,000 dollars required annually for tuition, not to mention room and board and other living expenses. His sisters Dee and Norma were in college now too, so the cumulative financial drain was enormous.

Returning from San Francisco, David felt confident that he would receive the loan. After all, his parents had built two churches for the denomination. David himself had served as president of the Northern Young People's Convention. And the Union was pouring thousands of dollars into low-cost housing for the poor. Surely they had an extra thousand dollars to lend a needy medical student who was considering going to the mission field as a doctor for the denomination.

Five days later David received a letter from the director of the Bay City Baptist Union. Eagerly he tore open the envelope, but his spirits plunged when he glimpsed the words, "We regret . . ."

Turned down! How could they do this to me! he stormed silently. His keen disappointment turned swiftly to anger, then bitterness. He felt shattered. He had been so sure that God would use the church to meet his financial need. He blamed the denominational leaders for their inconsistency, for having their priorities out of line, for neglecting their own. Stubbornly he resolved never again to have any association with the church.

When David explained his financial predicament to the university dean, the man observed wisely, "David, you are in the crucible of testing." He took a slow, deliberate breath and said, "I have a proposition to make. How would you like a scholarship to Quito, Ecuador?"

"Me—go to South America?" asked David in surprise. "How? When?"

"This summer. You'll assist a medical missionary. There's an 800 dollar stipend."

David hesitated. He removed his glasses and stared absently into space, his expression pinched. He had so recently resolved to have nothing more to do with the church. Now . . . to go to the mission field!

"I strongly urge you to go," said the dean, responding to David's obvious indecision. "I promise you that the experience will help you regain a perspective of God's calling."

Reluctantly David accepted the assignment. What choice did he have? He needed the money desperately.

But he received much more than money from his summer in Ecuador. He was blessed by the dedicated missionaries who took him to their hearts, and by the churches that embraced him with loving care and gratitude. As he confronted his own responsibility to humanity and to God, he found countless opportunities to share Christ and to minister to others.

Perhaps most important, as Christ dealt with him David lost his bitterness and self-pity. The lesson was clear. His Baptist brethren had not failed him; David himself had failed God. He had put his trust in an institution rather than in the Lord. He had allowed wounded pride and resentment to dictate his attitudes and behavior. Now he confessed his sins and sought forgiveness. He returned home with fresh appreciation for God's awesome lessons and resumed his participation in the local church.

After his return from Ecuador, David became even more romantically involved with Joyce. Being apart for the summer had been a lonely experience for both of them; the separation had only strengthened their mutual devotion. But being together again brought them face to face with a dilemma they could no longer ignore: the difference in their denominational backgrounds. Although David was attending an Adventist university, he had no intention of surrendering his Baptist heritage. Nor did Joyce feel she could marry anyone but an Adventist man.

For weeks David struggled with his conflicting feelings. Then one night he telephoned Joyce and told her they needed to talk. She agreed. He drove over with his good friend Oral Fisher, with whom he and Joyce had often double-dated. Oral respectfully left the two of them alone while he joined his own girl friend.

It was a disappointing evening for both David and Joyce.

They shared, cried, and embraced, knowing too well that the end of their relationship had come. "I love you beyond what I can describe," he told her, his voice breaking, "but I can't marry you. Our church differences would continually divide us."

"I know," she admitted gloomily. "I can't bend your way any more than you can bend mine."

Before going, he held her in his arms for one long, final moment. Their eyes met and lingered. With effort he broke away, said good-bye, and left quickly, without looking back.

Driving home that evening, David realized he had never felt such agony over the breakup of a romance. The misery obliterated everything—his thoughts, his reason . . . everything but the pain.

Oral sat beside him, trying to be reassuring. "Well, Dave," he murmured, "I wish I had words to say, but only you know what God wants for you."

David remained silent, his expression somber, his hands gripping the wheel. The dashboard clock said one A.M. He and Oral were on the San Bernardino Freeway, climbing to sixty . . . sixty-five miles per hour. Suddenly they came up behind another automobile traveling forty. David swerved vigorously to the left, but still the bumpers struck. The two cars caromed out of control. For an instant, the other vehicle looked as if it would turn over, but amazingly it did not.

The accident brought David abruptly out of his bitter reverie. He stopped with a jolt, jumped out, and checked the other car. He was greatly relieved to learn that the other driver, a sailor, was shaken but unhurt.

"I'm sorry. I didn't have my mind on my driving," David confessed. Looking at Oral he added miserably, "All I could see was Joyce."

In spite of his distress over losing Joyce, David made no effort to call her. In fact, they never saw each other again. Resolving to forget both Anglos and Adventists and get back where he "belonged," David threw himself wholeheartedly into the functions at the local Mexican Baptist church.

He still spent most of his time, day and night, studying. David had always been a conscientious student, but now he summoned even greater reserves of concentration and perseverance. He maintained a standard of excellence few of his classmates could match. But his unrelenting exertion took a physical and emotional toll.

Two months prior to his medical school graduation, David began to experience a strange inner turmoil. He was struck with bouts of unreasonable fear, emptiness, and insecurity. He felt dissatisfied. Distressingly, doubts about God bombarded him.

David was baffled. Why should he feel such a cloud of gloom? He had done well scholastically; bank loans had allowed him to keep his tuition payments current; and his cherished dream was about to reach fruition—he would be a doctor. Then why did he feel so doubtful, so depressed?

The more he pondered his peculiar state of restlessness and uncertainty, the more he felt like a hypocrite in God's universe. Was he attempting to be what he shouldn't and couldn't be? Had he manufactured a profession for himself to which he wasn't entitled?

David's doubts increased as final exams drew near. Then, perhaps prompted by the frantic pace of medical school, a persistent lack of sleep, and his nagging despondency, David developed a severe case of influenza. Lying in bed in his feverish, weakened condition, he sensed his despair growing. Startling questions plagued his disoriented mind. *Is God just a crutch . . . a means of escape . . . an ethereal Santa Claus . . . or perhaps a myth, a figment of my imagination?*

Desperate and driven by his quixotic introspection, David climbed out of bed at ten-thirty P.M., dressed, and began walking to the hospital a mile away. As he reached the entrance to the hospital, fear gripped him with such ferocity that he stopped, immobilized. *What was he doing here? What was happening to him?*

A public telephone booth near the hospital entrance caught his eye. Instinctively he walked over, stepped inside, and shut the door. The light failed to come on. Mechanically he picked up the receiver and dialed the operator. "I want to make a long distance call to San Jose," he said shakily, giving the number. Two . . . three rings, then his mother answered the phone. Hearing her voice, David began to cry.

His father picked up the extension phone and listened too as David blurted out his problem. "I am so confused, Mom . . . Dad. I'm ill . . . and I'm in doubt of God and his leading. A terrible fear is gripping me."

When he had finished, Margarita replied with unswerving conviction. "Son, God has chosen you for a great work. You are his! You have belonged to him since you accepted Jesus into your heart—remember? You were twelve. Now you must consider yourself an important participant in God's plan for the universe. He loves you, and we love you. Do you love him?"

Struggling to regain his composure, David replied, "Yes, Mom, I guess I do." His father prayed for him, a gentle, yearning prayer in Spanish. Afterward, David managed a faint thank you and good-bye.

For some time he remained in the dark phone booth, alone, praying while tears streamed down his face. He agonized with God, begging for a valid faith, for the Holy Spirit's power in his life. He felt Christ touching him, speaking, convicting. He thought about how he had been brought up in church; he had made a profession of faith and been baptized at the age of twelve. But not until now, at the age of twenty-five, while on the verge of completing his medical education, did David sense himself becoming integrated with Christ in a living, vital relationship. The doubts about God being a myth . . . a crutch . . . a figment of his imagination were erased—for good.

EIGHTEEN

In the fall of 1963, when David began his internship at White Memorial Medical Center in Los Angeles, his new spiritual commitment underwent immediate testing. His life-style changed dramatically. He experienced an over-whelming sense of emancipation, of personal and financial freedom. He had time on his hands; weekends were his own. No longer was he tied down by studies or restricted by a lack of funds. For the first time in his life he received a steady income—300 dollars a month, plus fifty dollars for every night of emergency room duty.

David's new freedom catapulted him into a vigorous routine of dating and partying. Over the past eight years he had been involved only with Ramona, and then Joyce. But now he enjoyed playing the field, lining up different dates for Friday, Saturday, and Sunday nights. Unwittingly he adopt-ed the "fun and games" attitude of many of the other interns. The question was not whether a girl was a Chris-tian, but rather, was she fun and attractive?

David's sportive, high-flown life-style culminated in an unsettling encounter with a glamorous Hollywood actress being featured in the movie, *The Interns*. David met her one. day at the hospital where the production crew was filming. They had lunch and dinner together at the hospital cafeteria. That weekend David asked her for a date.

But from the moment she stepped into his automobile, David felt an inexplicable oppressiveness of spirit. On a more practical level, he was irritated by the girl's chain-smoking. As he drove toward the Hollywood Bowl, he could not bear the growing sense of emptiness within him. Finally he pulled his car over to the curb, stopped, and looked woefully at the young lady. "You know, I have really made a mistake," he told her, the words catching in his throat. "You don't belong with me and I don't belong with you. We don't have a future together."

The girl stared back in stunned silence.

"Our cultural and religious backgrounds are totally different," continued David. "Even the little things like your chain-smoking . . . I don't smoke at all. So what are we doing together?" He paused, struggling to control his voice. "I know I've ruined your whole evening, but I—I think I'd better take you back home."

Coolly the young actress replied, "Fine . . . if that's the way you feel."

They drove home in silence, but the closer David got to her apartment to drop her off, the better he felt. He knew that he was doing the right thing.

That night David thought seriously about what his parents had always stressed—that he should seek his life partner from what they called "the family of God," and that there was no way to justify marrying outside of God's will. David prayed and promised the Lord that he would no longer date non-Christian girls. After that he began dating young ladies from the Pasadena and Alhambra First Baptist churches.

Then, early in 1964, David met Marilyn McLaughlin, a striking, vivacious blonde who had begun working as a clerk-secretary in the White Memorial emergency room. David noticed that Marilyn was the kind of gal a fellow looked twice at—physically appealing, with a bright, attractive personality, and popular with the guys. But first impressions told him she wasn't potential "wife and mother" material; she didn't seem to be the type who would be deeply committed to anything. So after brief but sober consideration, David concluded that he really was not attracted to Marilyn McLaughlin.

Nor was Marilyn McLaughlin particularly impressed by Dr. David Hernandez. She first heard his name mentioned while waiting for an orientation meeting to begin in the White emergency room. Several nurses and secretaries sat talking about "that cute Dr. Hernandez." One girl prattled, "Oh, he's so friendly with everyone ... especially the nurses. And just think, he's single!" But Marilyn paid little attention to their conversation. She wasn't about to be impressed by any intern. Why, some of them were egotistical, opinionated boors!

A few days later, as Marilyn and her roommate were walking near the hospital, the girl pointed across the street at a slender young man in glasses and a white jacket and said, "There's that Filipino doctor, Dr. Hernandez."

Marilyn looked over without concern and mused silently, "He looks Mexican to me, but maybe there's not that much difference."

Often after that she saw Dr. Hernandez in the emergency room. She noted that he had a way of walking through and not really saying anything, but making it obvious that he was there. He had an impeccable reputation as an intern, but Marilyn imagined him to be a most conceited, overbearing man.

One night after completing her three-to-eleven P.M. shift, Marilyn began walking to her apartment a block and a half from the hospital. Without warning, a car pulled over beside her and stopped. Dr. Hernandez rolled down his window and asked, "Would you like a ride?"

"No thanks," replied Marilyn in a small, startled voice. "I just live around the corner." She continued walking.

David followed slowly beside her. "But I'm going down that way," he persisted. "Don't you want a ride?"

"No," she said again. It seemed silly to accept a ride when she lived so close.

"Why not?" said David, irritation stealing into his voice. "I'm visiting a friend right around the corner."

Marilyn's discomfiture was growing. "But I'm almost there."

"OK, have it your way," snapped David, pulling away in a huff. He sped around the corner, and Marilyn assumed that was that—until they met again minutes later. Coincidentally the doctor's appointment was in the apartment just above hers. It was evident in their cool exchange of greetings that they had made quite an impression on each other—one that was unquestionably negative.

But on New Year's Eve, Marilyn's attitude toward David Hernandez changed incontrovertibly. She had completed her three-to-eleven shift, gone home and changed into slacks, then returned to the emergency room to meet some friends. One of the nurses had arranged a blind date for Marilyn with her fiancé's best buddy. While waiting, Marilyn sat down at the desk and began catching up on some office work.

It was nearly midnight when David ambled into the room and sat down on the desk where she was working. "Well, things look pretty quiet around here," he remarked.

Marilyn glanced up briefly and nodded.

"Up until midnight," he continued, "people are at parties or concerts or somewhere. But after two or three in the morning, then it will get rough."

Again she nodded.

"I'm on call until seven A.M., but your shift ended at eleven. So how come you're still puttering around here?"

Marilyn was about to answer, but suddenly horns began sounding outside and fireworks exploded in the distance. It was midnight, the beginning of a new year. David leaned over and asked suavely, "Do you mind if I kiss you?"

Marilyn looked up in surprise and murmured, "No, I don't mind." It wasn't just a peck on the cheek, but a firm kiss on the mouth, tender, lingering. Marilyn would never forget it.

Five minutes later she left with the engaged couple and her blind date. They drove to Long Beach, stopped for a bite to eat, then walked along the beach.

Marilyn noticed with alarm that the other couple had stopped to kiss. She glanced at her date—a nice enough guy but virtually a stranger—and knew she didn't want to get into a compromising situation with him. Besides, David's kiss was still fresh on her lips. It had been surprisingly special. She didn't want to erase the memory of it now.

So she kicked off her shoes, rolled up her pant legs, and

waded out into the water. It was uncomfortably cold, but she stood there for twenty minutes, waiting. Her toes began to ache, and gradually the pain crept into her feet and legs as well, but she refused to move. Her date, in expensive slacks and shoes, remained on shore, silently perplexed. When he called irritably, "Marilyn, when are you coming out of that water?" she chattered back, "I—I l-like it here."

Finally, after what seemed like hours, the engaged couple returned to the car, followed by a numb, thoroughly chilled Marilyn and her disgruntled companion.

They dropped Marilyn off first. She shivered her way out of the car and into the house. Her friends roared off in evident relief. In spite of her immense discomfort, Marilyn still found herself thinking fondly of David Hernandez and his unexpected kiss.

Following that evening, David and Marilyn developed a pleasant working relationship in the emergency room. They joked around together and chatted amiably. Marilyn was convinced now that she had misjudged David. He was a lot of fun, not at all stuffy and insufferable as she had originally supposed.

Then one day he asked her for a date. She quickly accepted. They went to see *The Sound of Music.* Afterward, they talked. David asked Marilyn if she was a Christian.

"Yes, of course I'm a Christian," she replied, surprised. Silently she wondered, *What's a Christian?* She reasoned that she was a good person; she *tried* to be a good person. Certainly she wasn't a heathen, so didn't that make her a Christian?

"What church do you attend?" questioned David.

"Church?"

"Yes, what denomination are you? You know, Baptist . . . Methodist—?"

"Oh, I'm Methodist," replied Marilyn firmly. She recalled that her sister Charlene had been married in a Methodist church. It was the one time Marilyn had been inside a church, so didn't that make her a Methodist?

David smiled uncertainly. "Well, maybe you'd like to go to church with me sometime."

Over the next six months David and Marilyn's dates were

limited to occasional tennis matches at a nearby park. Nearly every week he asked her if she had attended church on Sunday. Then he would ask her what the sermon was about. In self-defense Marilyn began attending a nearby Methodist church. She faithfully saved every bulletin to prove to David that she had been in church. It was a peculiar sort of game; but if David wanted her in church, then to church she would go. Now and then he invited her to join him at the Alhambra First Baptist Church. Marilyn went, eager for any opportunity to be with him.

While Marilyn enjoyed her random church and tennis dates with David, she was particularly pleased when he took her somewhere special—to a formal concert, a play, a fancy restaurant. But one summer evening became a near social calamity for Marilyn. She was dressing for dinner, slipping into her best outfit—a lovely, black, sleeveless dress—when the back zipper broke. David was due to arrive any moment and Marilyn had nothing else to wear. On impulse, she decided to hide her dilemma beneath her stylish leopard coat.

Marilyn's strategy might have proved less of a fiasco had the weather not been so unbearably hot. When they arrived at the restaurant—a warm, closed building without air-conditioning—David offered to take her coat. Marilyn defensively pulled it tighter around her and said, "No thanks. I'll wear it." At the table, David again politely suggested she take off her coat.

"Oh, no," replied Marilyn with a forced smile. "I'm really very cool."

As he stared curiously at her, she realized her face was beading with perspiration. She struggled through the meal, melting, slowly dying inside, trying her best to maintain a favorable impression. One last time David urged her to remove her coat, but Marilyn was adamant; the coat stayed on.

Finally he shook his head and mumbled under his breath, "Weird. She just won't take that thing off."

It would be many years before Marilyn would find the courage to reveal to David her reason for refusing to remove her leopard coat.

During David's second year of residency, Marilyn gave up her apartment and moved back home temporarily. Her parents, Laurence and Bevan McLaughlin, knew that she was dating a Mexican resident physician, but they hadn't met him yet. Marilyn was sure they would like him. The McLaughlins were kind, open, unpretentious people who entertained no prejudices.

It was true, however, that when Marilyn had first started seeing David, her mother had remarked, "Why don't you let him date Mexican girls and you just date Anglos?"

Marilyn had replied blithely, "Don't panic, Mom. I'm not going to marry the guy."

But now that Marilyn's feelings for David were growing, both her parents offered only their support and encouragement.

So now it was time for them to meet David. One weekend when he asked her out, she told him she wanted him to meet her parents. He agreed to make it that night when he picked her up.

That evening Marilyn felt as if she were getting ready for her first date. The house had to be spotless, everything perfect. Just before David was due to arrive, Marilyn scooped up the family pet, Yankee, a large old Siamese cat, and hugged him. "Mom, I'm as jumpy as this cat," she said, laughing. The animal wriggled out of her arms and sprang to the floor. "Say, Mom, does he still get in as many cat fights as he used to?" she asked offhandedly.

"Not anymore," replied her mother with a sly gleam. "See that red plastic horn on the table by the sofa? It makes a terrible, unearthly sound. Whenever I hear a cat fight, I go out and blow that horn and it scares all the other cats away. Our Yankee knows he's been rescued."

"Great idea," said Marilyn. She glanced nervously at the clock. Seven P.M. Moments later she heard a car pull up out front. "Mom! Dad! He's here," she called. "Look at his big new car. A Grand Prix. Isn't it beautiful?" She gazed excitedly at her parents and whispered, "I want so much for us to make a good impression."

Introductions went well. David was gallant and polite; her parents were warm and natural. Everyone sat down for a few minutes to talk. At last David said, "Mr. and Mrs. McLaughlin, in my home when my sisters went out on a date, my dad always insisted that they be home by a certain time. So what time would you like Marilyn to be home?"

Marilyn's mother smiled pleasantly and said, "I would like to have her back by eleven."

"Eleven?" repeated David in surprise.

Eleven! echoed Marilyn silently. Was her mother kidding? Marilyn was twenty-one and had already lived on her own. Eleven had to be a joke. But there wasn't the slightest hint of humor in her mother's expression.

There was a lengthy pause. Then, retrieving his voice and his poise, David said, "Fine. She'll be home by eleven."

For an instant Marilyn had an impulse to throw something. But she wasn't sure whom she wished more to hit—David or her mother.

The foursome chatted some more; light, casual conversation. Then suddenly, in mid-sentence, Marilyn's mother jumped up from her place on the sofa, grabbed the red plastic horn, and ran out onto the front porch. There was a hideous, ear-splitting sound, accompanied by the spit-snarl of several cats. Mrs. McLaughlin came back inside, shut the door, and with a grand smile of satisfaction returned the horn to its spot on the table. With scarcely a pause and no explanation, she calmly resumed the conversation where she had left off.

"Cat fight," Marilyn inserted in red-faced embarrassment. But it was obvious from David's startled, incredulous expression that he had no idea what she was talking about, and no possible conception of what had just taken place. Without a doubt Marilyn had got her wish. Her parents had made an unforgettable—if unorthodox—impression on Dr. David Hernandez.

But David's impression of Marilyn wasn't dampened in the least. Shortly after they had dated steadily for three weekends in a row, she received an unexpected telephone call from him. She was at her desk in the emergency room; he was calling from a music store in Pasadena. He said, "I just can't make up my mind between these two records." He named the albums and asked, "Which do you think I should buy?"

Marilyn was immensely pleased that David had bothered to call for her opinion. It was such a sweet, impulsive thing for him to do—so unlike the cautious, conservative David she knew. "I really don't know what to tell you," she said, laughing, feeling flattered and flustered at once. "You know, pick out whichever one you want."

Unexpectedly he whispered, "I love you."

"What?" she asked in astonishment.

"I love you," he said again.

"No, you don't. You're just infatuated."

"Don't tell me that. I really love you."

Marilyn tried in vain to remain calm. "Oh, you don't," she said again, more softly, not really trying to convince him. In her heart she knew he didn't really love her, not yet. But infatuation was enough for now. For her, there was no longer a question about how she felt. She cared deeply for David. It was a slowly growing, inevitable love, one she hoped someday he would feel in turn.

NINETEEN

David was in a dilemma. He and Marilyn had been dating casually, off and on, for over two years now. But their relationship raised more questions than it answered. Did David love Marilyn? Did they have a future together? Did God approve of their relationship? Distressingly, David wasn't even sure Marilyn was a Christian. Of course, she regularly attended church and single young adult activities with him, but he doubted that she had ever made a personal commitment to Christ. That would mean he was going back on his promise to God. As long as the disturbing question of Marilyn's salvation remained unanswered, David could not entertain serious intentions toward her. But then, was he callously leading Marilyn on by dating her?

There was the question, too, of David's parents. What would they think if he brought home a blonde Anglo girl? He could answer that question all too easily. Mom would be furious. She would insist, "You should marry a nice Mexican girl, your own kind!"

Another issue, at least in David's own mind, was Marilyn's health. She was diabetic. It wasn't a problem now, but if they married, what complications in her health might they face in later years? And what about the effect on their children? As a physician, David could not lightly dismiss such concerns.

It was likely that David had not confronted these issues sooner because he had little desire to get serious with any girl. True, he was nearly thirty, but David, like many of his friends, was not ready to commit himself. He liked his freedom. His life was pleasant, fulfilling. He had a busy, stimulating career in medicine, and he spent most of his free hours working with the young people at church. So why take a chance of ruining everything with marriage, an unknown—and presently unnecessary—factor?

But David could no longer ignore the fact that Marilyn was looking for commitment, a relationship with a future. To play games with her emotions wasn't healthy for either of them.

Then, early in January 1967, there was a significant turn of events. Following an evening evangelistic service, Marilyn made a personal profession of faith in Christ. Both David and Marilyn rejoiced in this new dimension of sharing in their lives. Now that the primary obstacle to their relationship was eliminated, David felt a new urgency to evaluate their possible future together.

But the more he analyzed, the more pressured both he and Marilyn felt. They found themselves bickering frequently, at odds emotionally. They had always had their share of differences, of course. David lived essentially by his intellect, Marilyn by her heart. Their backgrounds, attitudes, and personalities were vastly different.

Marilyn was especially irritated by David's habit of taking her to a church party or other function and disappearing into the crowd, only to rejoin her hours later when it was time to leave. "In high school when a guy took me to a party, he didn't just dump me," she told David time and again. "We spent the evening together."

But the more Marilyn protested, the more aggravated David became. He loved mixing with people, making new acquaintances. Why didn't Marilyn feel that way? He figured if she had enough going for her, she would enjoy other people; she would want to stand on her own two feet rather than hang on his arm all evening.

Gradually David began to realize that he wasn't giving Marilyn the consideration she deserved; he wasn't allowing her to be herself. It struck him disconcertingly one day, *I want her to be me!* Once he caught that insight into himself, he made an effort to be more sensitive to Marilyn's needs.

But David was totally unprepared for the crisis that erupted between the two of them one evening late in January. It started out as a routine date, except that Marilyn seemed a bit edgy and quieter than usual. David, his arm lightly around Marilyn's shoulder, made an offhand remark about how they had a lot going for them.

Without warning, Marilyn stiffened and pulled away. "No, David," she said sharply, "we don't have anything going for us."

David sat forward and stared at her. "What do you mean by that?"

Marilyn's voice was tremulous. "I've finally gotten myself to the place where I can say this. We have been going together for so long, but we're getting nowhere fast." She looked at him, her eyes welling with tears. "You've never even taken me to meet your folks. I don't know anything about your family or your background. We argue more than we get along. These last couple years have been one long frustration for me, and it's not getting any better."

"Marilyn, I—I didn't realize—" said David, groping for words.

"It's over, David," she said, cutting him off. "This is the end; there's nothing more." Her voice faltered momentarily, and she looked away. "Don't call me; don't come over. Let's just break it off here." She began to cry.

David reached out to comfort her. "Is it because I haven't mentioned marriage?"

"Marriage?" scoffed Marilyn, dabbing at her tears. "With our backgrounds so different, even if we got married it wouldn't work out."

David suddenly found himself weeping too. "What do you want me to do, hon?"

"Go away. I don't want to talk about it anymore."

David left then, dazed, radically shaken. He went home and prayed earnestly. He had to decide once and for all how he really felt about Marilyn. Did he love her? Would he love her forever? Was he prepared to spend a lifetime with her? If not, he would have to leave her alone for good.

David felt too confused, too unsettled to rely on his emotions. Somehow he had to see things in perspective, plainly, in black and white. In medicine, when he needed an answer he applied the scientific method. So he decided now to make a list, to get something down on paper. Pros and cons, both his and Marilyn's negative and positive traits, their virtues, their faults. He put down everything he could think of. He found his own "negative" list surprisingly long. He compared the lists, determining how his positive traits would complement hers, how his faults might distress her.

When he had finished, he sat back and marveled. "There really is some logic to this thing," he said aloud. "Our relationship is solid. It's not all just feelings or friendship or physical attraction. I really do love her."

David telephoned Marilyn the next day, but she refused to talk. He called several times the following week, but she wouldn't see him.

Finally, in desperation David telephoned Marilyn's mother. In a calm, formal voice he announced, "I am in a situation right now where I feel that I want to make a serious commitment to Marilyn. You may think this is childish that I should call you, but I don't think so. I feel like I should tell you that I do love your daughter, and I have reached the point where I am no longer playing games. I've given every aspect of our relationship serious consideration, including the fact that Marilyn is diabetic; and I've overcome any personal doubts I might have had." He caught his breath and rushed on before she could reply. "I haven't seen Marilyn for a few days. We're having a conflict and she prefers that I don't see her. But perhaps you can tell her I really am serious about her."

"I appreciate your calling me, David," replied Mrs. McLaughlin pleasantly. "I haven't seen Marilyn for a few days either, but when she calls I'll reassure her about you."

A few days later, when he had received no word from Mrs. McLaughlin, David tried once more to communicate his feelings to Marilyn. "Please, honey," he urged over the telephone, "let's give it another try. I really do feel we have a future together."

This time Marilyn was willing to talk. "Come over, David," she said. "I have something to tell you too."

Shortly after his arrival, Marilyn explained her change of heart. "I prayed about our relationship, David," she said. "It was a hard thing for me because I knew what I wanted, but I had this fatalistic attitude . . . like I haven't been a Christian long enough, and you've been a Christian all these years. I've made many stupid mistakes, and I know so little about the Bible. I figured I could never be the kind of wife you want me to be. I felt that our being together was the last thing the Lord wanted for us."

"That's not true," interrupted David.

"Wait, there's more," she said quickly. "That's when I felt I should pray about it. I'd never really prayed about something like this; it was kind of new to me. But I prayed and prayed. And, David, I got this tremendous peace . . . something I never experienced before . . . like what the Bible calls the peace that passes all understanding. Not just peace, but an assurance that I really could make you happy. I realized that things are going to be OK. The Lord really is with us."

Wordlessly they embraced. Then David whispered, "God has truly given us a fresh beginning."

The next day David telephoned Marilyn at the Department of Water and Power, where she was working. He asked if he could drive her to her class that evening at California Baptist Theological Seminary in Pomona.

"No, its really not necessary," she replied.

"Please," urged David. "We still have many things to settle between us."

"All right," said Marilyn, relenting.

That night David pulled into the campus parking lot, turned off the motor, and looked over at Marilyn. The moon shone through the window, illuminating her face with a fine, silvery glow. A romantic ballad wafted from the car radio. "Honey," said David, "before you go into class, I want to tell you something." He reached out for her hand and rubbed it gently. "Babe, I want you to marry me."

"Oh, David," replied Marilyn softly, "I want that too, but how can we talk about it now? I have to get in to class."

"Okay, we'll continue this later tonight," he agreed.

David walked Marilyn to her class and remained for the session. Afterward they drove to a nearby restaurant where they talked more than they ate.

For the first time, David felt himself truly opening up to Marilyn, sharing some of his innermost thoughts and concerns. "God has to be first in my life," he said earnestly. "No one else can be first, not even you or my parents."

Marilyn nodded, but David wasn't sure she understood. "I say this," he continued, "because there are times that I get the feeling from you that you get aggravated because I spend too much time with church activities. I want this absolutely clear now that God *must* be first in my life."

"Yes, I know," said Marilyn, nodding again.

"And you would be second in my life," David explained. "Would you be able to accept that kind of relationship?"

"What do you really mean by that?" she asked uncertainly. "Does it mean that I get neglected?"

"No, it doesn't mean neglecting you at all," said David. "But it does mean that God has priority. There may be times when you think I'm committing myself too much to religious things, and you may feel you are taking second place. But that's the way it has to be."

"It's a new idea to me," Marilyn admitted. "In my family my parents have always come first with each other."

"Well, if you don't think God can have first place," cautioned David, "then we can't make a go of it."

Thoughtfully Marilyn turned the handle of her coffee mug. They had sat talking for so long that the coffee was cold. She looked up at David and said, "No, it seems like a good idea, God coming first. I want to marry you, David, and I feel that God has given me the go-ahead." She smiled warmly, her green eyes glistening. "If I have to take second place, God isn't such a bad one to follow."

"Then I think we've got everything settled," said David,

returning her smile. "How do you think your folks will feel about us?"

Marilyn laughed lightly. "Well, we've dated for so long, Mom wonders if we're ever going to get married. But seriously, I talked to her and she told me about your phone call. She knows I love you, and she says she and Daddy will love you as much as I do."

"That's great," said David. He sipped his coffee, then replaced the cup in a slow, deliberate gesture. "Now I think it's about time for you to meet my parents. What would you think of driving up to San Jose with me one weekend soon?"

Marilyn couldn't hide her excitement. "Oh, David, I'd love it," she cried. "I'd absolutely love it!"

PART FIVE
DAVID
AND MARILYN
HERNANDEZ

TWENTY

We're on our way to San Jose. Marilyn couldn't believe how perfect everything was working out. David had actually proposed marriage and now she was on her way to meet his folks.

How she had waited to get acquainted with his family. She loved David so much. She wanted that love to spill over to everyone who was part of David. She wanted it to be as it was with Ruth in the Bible: "Your people shall be my people."

David confirmed Marilyn's optimism. "You'll like my parents," he assured her. "They're plain, humble Christians. They love people. In fact, they always have a houseful of guests—church folk, kids who need a helping hand. And Mom is a real treasure, so friendly and outgoing. You'll love her."

It was a Friday evening. David and Marilyn were riding up to San Jose with David's sister Norma, her husband Willie, and their baby daughter Denise. They pulled into the Hernandez driveway at ten P.M. As they piled out of the automobile, Margarita Hernandez came running outside to greet them. Without a glance at Marilyn, she took baby Denise in her arms. As everyone entered the house, there was a flurry of greetings and introductions—David's parents, his sister Dee, his Grandfather Jesus. But afterward Marilyn couldn't recall that David's mother had even spoken to her. Shortly Dee, an attractive girl in her mid-twenties, led Marilyn to a bedroom and said, "You'll be sharing this room with Norma and me."

"I have some candy for your mother," Marilyn said timidly. "Would you give it to her?"

"Oh, no, you give it to her," Dee said brightly. She left the room momentarily and returned with her mother. Gingerly Marilyn handed Margarita the candy.

"I don't know why everybody brings me candy when they come to visit," replied Margarita with a crisp, slightly accusing laugh.

"Well, I hope you enjoy it," said Marilyn lamely. Inexplicably, she felt terrified inside. Without another word Margarita turned and left the room.

The next morning when Marilyn approached the breakfast table, she prayed that her first impressions were wrong. Surely David's mother didn't dislike her as much as she sensed. Marilyn had come here as David's future wife. He expected her to fit in. This was supposed to be a warm, wonderful beginning. More than anything, Marilyn wanted his family to like her.

But Margarita's first words directly to her that morning were, "Do you know how much I have sacrificed for this boy" (nodding toward David in the other room) "what I have given up to put him through school?"

Her words petrified Marilyn. She didn't know how to respond. She mumbled something unintelligible, then quickly sat down at the table. Margarita remained stonily silent through breakfast. Jose Hernandez, a quiet man by nature, interjected an occasional comment, and Dee and Norma chatted amiably. But Marilyn ate without a word, precariously close to tears.

After breakfast, David said with forced animation, "Who wants to go in to San Francisco with Marilyn and me?"

"I'd better stay home with Denise," said Norma.

"No, thanks, son," said Jose.

"Not me. I've got too much to do," said Margarita sharply.

David's enthusiasm dissolved. "Well, you folks can stay here . . . but if anyone wants to join us . . ."

"I'll go," said Dee, glancing uneasily from her mother to Marilyn.

"Me, too," said David's Grandfather Jesus with a solemn nod.

Later, as they approached the crowded, glistening city, Marilyn asked David tentatively, "What did you tell your parents about me?"

"Nothing," he replied.

"Nothing? You didn't tell them we're getting married?"

"No. But I will . . . soon." He gazed questioningly at her. "Tell me, Babe, are you having a good time?"

"Oh, yes," said Marilyn, forcing a smile. "I'm having a wonderful time. Your folks are very . . . nice."

In spite of their unspoken misgivings, David and Marilyn had marvelous fun with Dee and Grandfather Jesus in San Francisco. They visited Fisherman's Wharf, strolled leisurely through Chinatown, and rode the cable cars over weaving hill-and-gully streets. But when they returned to the Hernandez home, Marilyn sensed the same repelling chill. Margarita Hernandez refused to speak to her.

That evening Dee remarked that she and a friend were going to the drugstore. Did anyone want anything?

"I'd like to go along," said Marilyn quickly.

She rode with the girls downtown. But while they went to the drugstore, Marilyn found a public phone booth and telephoned her roommate Diane in Los Angeles.

"So how's everything going?" asked Diane eagerly. "I hope you're in seventh heaven up there with David and his family."

Marilyn burst into tears. "Oh, Diane, they hate me," she sobbed. "It's a complete disaster. His folks won't even talk to me. Why didn't David tell me it would be like this? Why didn't he warn me?"

"Listen, Marilyn," said Diane. "You go back there and be your own sweet self. If they want to be mean, that's their problem. I'll admit, I was afraid it would be like this, but just hang in there. Don't let it wreck things between you and David."

"But I—I've never been so miserable in my life. And I can't even let David know how I feel. He acts like everything's just fine!"

After several minutes Marilyn composed herself, hung up the phone, and joined Dee for the drive back to the house.

On Sunday, just before David and Marilyn were scheduled to fly back to Los Angeles, Jose Hernandez sat down beside Marilyn and asked, "How long have you been a Christian?"

"Actually, just a few weeks," said Marilyn earnestly. "I'm a new Christian, but I really love the Lord."

"What church do you go to?"

"The same Baptist church that David attends."

Jose smiled and nodded. That was the extent of their conversation. But Marilyn felt overjoyed that David's father had even bothered to speak to her.

On the flight back that evening, David and Marilyn sat in separate worlds of silence, both absorbed in their own private, painful reveries. David felt strung out, caught in the middle, torn between his loyalty to his parents and his love for Marilyn. His mind was in flux. He had supposed he had resolved his doubts about Marilyn. The two of them had just come through their own turbulent crisis; but now, unexpectedly, he was thrown into greater turmoil than ever. He should have known how his parents would react to Marilyn—an Anglo, a new Christian, a stranger. They were still pulling for Ramona, hoping against hope that David would decide to marry her. But for David, that matter had been settled long ago. Now there was only Marilyn.

David glanced over at his future bride. He knew the weekend hadn't been easy for her. Marilyn was a sweet, vulnerable girl. Surely she had been hurt by the cold reception she received. He realized he ought to offer comfort, reassurance. But how could he, when he himself felt so ambivalent? His feelings fluctuated between intense aggravation at his folks for refusing to understand his position, and a sort of obscure anger at Marilyn for unknowingly placing him in the middle between her and his parents.

Perhaps most of all, he felt bitterly disappointed. He had always had great respect for his parents and their opinions. He had been brought up to believe that disobeying one's parents was almost as bad as rejecting God's Word. Now he was suddenly thrust into a volatile situation where it appeared he could be guilty of just such disobedience.

But he was a grown man, nearly thirty years old. Surely selecting a life partner should be his own choice, his responsibility, a matter between him and God. But what if he were wrong about Marilyn, about their future together? The idea gnawed at him, *If you are wrong, you'll pay the price for it. And tragically, so will Marilyn.*

David glanced again at Marilyn. Their eyes met and held. "Well, it was quite a weekend, wasn't it?" he said with brisk cheerfulness.

"Yes," replied Marilyn, offering a thin smile. "Quite a weekend!"

Nothing else was said about their undeniably bizarre trip to San Jose. But the weekend had been a shattering experience for both David and Marilyn. In fact, six months passed before either of them mentioned another word about their engagement. Only once was the subject indirectly broached, and that was by Marilyn's roommate shortly after the trip.

"Has David said anything yet about a ring?" she asked Marilyn.

"No, nothing at all."

"Well, why don't you tell me what style you want, and I'll call David and tell him I'll be happy to help him pick one out."

It seemed like a good idea. But when Diane telephoned David, he dismissed her idea with a curt reply. "Oh, I have everything under control," he said. "I think I know what she wants."

Marilyn waited and waited. Spring passed and summer arrived. David completed his three-year post-graduate residency in obstetrics and gynecology at White Memorial Medical Center, plus six months rotation at Rancho Los Amigos, Los Angeles County Hospital, in Downey. David had decided on the field of obstetrics because he believed so strongly in the importance of the home; he wanted the opportunity to help families. He especially wanted to be available in his practice to help families in the Mexican-American community. Obstetrics would also give him a good balance between surgery and office practice. And he would be dealing with a nice, generally healthy segment of the population—not the very young, as in pediatrics, nor the very old, as in geriatrics.

As the fall of 1967 approached, David received his draft

notice from the U. S. Army. He was ordered to report to Fort Sam Houston in San Antonio, Texas, for the two-month Medical Basic Course. His permanent duty station would be at Fort Carson, Colorado, where he would serve in the OB-GYN Section of the U. S. Army Hospital.

On Monday, September 6, five days before David was due at "Fort Sam," he told Marilyn, "You know, Babe, I'm leaving for Texas in two days. Don't you think maybe we should go get you an engagement ring?"

Don't I think! Marilyn wanted to shout. Instead, she said sweetly, "Oh, David, that would be wonderful!"

That very afternoon David and Marilyn visited a friend of his who was a jeweler, to pick out a ring. "This will be ready for you by noon on Wednesday," he told them when they had made their selection.

Wednesday, September 8, was an incredibly busy day. David and Marilyn spent the morning in his second-story apartment packing boxes and crates for the moving van. At eleven-thirty, when David had mentioned nothing about the engagement ring, Marilyn said tentatively, "It's about noon, David. Maybe we should go get the ring."

"Oh, that's right," he said as if it were a novel idea. He left her in charge of the packing while he drove over to the jeweler's. But when he returned a short time later, he mentioned nothing about the ring.

"David, where is it?" Marilyn asked, trying to contain her eagerness.

"It's down in the glove compartment," he replied nonchalantly. "Why don't you go down and get it?"

Marilyn didn't have to be told twice. She ran downstairs, while David followed at what seemed a snail's pace. They sat together in the car. He slipped the ring on her finger, and they kissed for one long tender moment.

Then David sat back and said, "You know, I'm really hungry. Why don't you go over to the Orange Julius and get us some hamburgers?"

Marilyn was too dazzled to argue—or to bother David for the money for the food. Obediently she went after the hamburgers. As she waited for her order, she was amazed that no one noticed the magnificent diamond gleaming on her finger.

That evening David and Marilyn went to his sister Norma's home for a "going-away" dinner—and an unofficial engagement party. David's parents and his Grandmother Sabina flew in from San Jose to see him off. David would be leaving at midnight, taking his grandmother with him as far as Phoenix, where she would be visiting relatives.

Norma's farewell dinner presented Marilyn with her second encounter with David's parents. She had no idea whether they knew of their son's engagement. David had not mentioned his folks since their unfortunate trip to San Jose nearly seven months before. She assumed he had said nothing to them about her either.

The dinner was superb, but Marilyn felt too apprehensive to say a word to anyone. David glanced nervously at Marilyn, at her ring, then at his parents. They didn't seem to notice the stone glistening on her finger.

Margarita Hernandez was clearly emotional about her son being drafted. "David, you've been away from us for a long time," she said sadly, "but now it seems like you are really leaving us."

While everyone still sat around the table, Jose Hernandez stood up, bowed his head, and, in Spanish, offered a lengthy prayer for his son. Marilyn shifted uneasily. Everyone else knew what he was saying, but she couldn't understand a word.

After the prayer, Norma spoke up. "Marilyn, don't you have something to show us?"

Marilyn looked entreatingly at David. He looked back with a strange, startled expression, as if he might be about to choke. Marilyn had a fleeting sensation that he wished he could slide unobtrusively under the table. She herself felt ready to bolt for the nearest door.

"Get on with it, brother," laughed Norma, holding up Marilyn's hand for everyone to see. "Now's the time."

For a moment no one spoke. The tension in the room was razor-sharp. Finally David said in a low, tight voice, "Yes, I wanted to show the family the ring."

Dee came over and examined the ring, then Marilyn extended her hand nervously to the rest of the family. There were enthusiastic words of congratulations and exclamations of "Oh, how beautiful!" But what Marilyn couldn't miss was Margarita Hernandez craning her neck slightly to see the ring, then turning away wordlessly, her expression lined with disapproval.

The ring was forgotten temporarily as midnight approached and the family gathered around David to say good-bye.

In the flurry of farewells, David embraced Marilyn and said with faltering voice, "I don't know exactly when we'll get married, Babe. I mean, I'll have to fly home. It'll be on my first leave—maybe November or December or even January."

"I'll be here waiting, whenever it is," whispered Marilyn, fighting back tears. "I love you."

"I love you too," he said, giving her one last hug.

On October 15, 1967, David notified Marilyn that he would be granted ten days leave late in November. She would have little more than a month to make arrangements for their wedding.

On November 4, David sent a letter to Marilyn's parents, officially announcing his plans to marry their daughter. The letter was typewritten, excessively formal, and signed "David Hernandez, M.D." He said in part, "We feel our love is well-rooted, nurtured in a mature fashion, and the decision has followed bilateral scrutiny of our motives. For this reason we have made the decision to concretize our love in marriage at the First Baptist Church of Alhambra the 26th of November at two P.M."

Mrs. McLaughlin replied with a brief, friendly letter. Speaking of the upcoming wedding, she said, "Marilyn is excited and tense and I am too, I suppose. We both snap at each other now and then. I understand, and I truly hope that she does. . . . Marilyn is so anxious to be with you, and in her new home. . . . I know that you and Marilyn will have a wonderful life together. She is a lovely girl, and she loves and misses her David very much."

But while Marilyn's parents looked forward to the marriage, David's folks were anything but enthusiastic. In a telephone conversation, David learned from his sister Norma that his mother was not planning to come to the wedding. In a quiet, controlled voice, he told Norma, "When you see Dad, tell him I would appreciate it if *he* showed up."

Later David himself talked with his father on the phone. Jose told him, "Son, don't worry about it. We will show up. Even though your mother has threatened not to come, I know at the last minute she will be there . . . because she loves you."

David wasn't so convinced, but he didn't want to worry Marilyn, so he kept the problem to himself. He flew home five days before the wedding. They were married by Dr. Harold Sweezey on Sunday, November 26. Both sets of parents were there, although Margarita remained cool and reserved.

David, feeling more nervous than he had ever been in his life, faltered slightly in repeating his vows, which managed to strike momentary terror in Marilyn's heart. Otherwise the ceremony went well, and in a few brief minutes David and Marilyn became Dr. and Mrs. David Hernandez.

That evening they left in Marilyn's Volkswagen for Colorado Springs, where they would live in a little apartment five miles north of the base. Since David had to check in on Thursday morning, their honeymoon consisted of their three-day drive to Colorado. It was not an impressive honeymoon, but both David and Marilyn agreed: the best thing for both of them was to be together, away from their families. For the first time ever they were totally, blissfully on their own.

TWENTY-ONE

David and Marilyn had been married only three months when they received an early morning telephone call from David's mother. On impulse she had driven to Colorado Springs for a visit. Now she was in town, just minutes away, and needed directions to their rented apartment. Marilyn was aghast. It wasn't possible. People didn't do such things—make a three-day trip and drop in without warning or an invitation!

"I'd be glad to have her visit," Marilyn told David in a slightly dazed, hysterical voice, "if I had time to plan and prepare. How can she just show up on our doorstep like this?"

"That's Mom," said David with a shrug. "At least she called first."

"Great!" wailed Marilyn. "We have a half-hour notice. The house is a mess, we have absolutely no food, and you don't get paid until next week. She'll think we're starving to death."

"We'll manage," said David reassuringly. He glanced into the refrigerator. "Look, we have that tongue in the freezer that you bought for me at the PX."

"That's still there because I don't know how to fix it," she retorted. "What am I supposed to do? Set this gigantic frozen tongue on the table for dinner?"

"That's not a bad idea," mused David.

"What?"

"Mom likes tongue. She knows how to fix it."

"Well, how long is she staying? Did she say?"

"No, probably only a few days . . . or maybe a couple of weeks."

"How will we entertain her?" asked Marilyn, taking a dust cloth from the drawer. "You work every day at the base, and I have my job at the clinic."

"Mom will amuse herself," said David with a confident smile.

"But if only I had some time to make things special for her," said Marilyn, swiftly dusting one table, then another.

"That's Mexican culture for you," said David, laughing. "Like I've said before, when I was growing up our house was like Grand Central Station. Hundreds of young people received love, food, and shelter in our home. Seminary students from Mexico, Guatemala, and Costa Rica, having no relatives in this country, would show up and spend Christmas vacation with us. Sometimes a carload of kids from the church or seminary would appear at the door. My folks would spread out the mattresses on the floor, hand out blankets, and make the beans go as far as possible. Mom would get up at two in the morning to make tortillas for the crowd."

"Well, I'm not your mother," Marilyn responded curtly, "and my parents' home wasn't like yours. Right now I need your help to get ready for just one unexpected lady."

For all the distress and confusion of that morning, Margarita Hernandez' visit turned out much better than anyone anticipated. Apparently Margarita had resolved her antagonism toward the marriage, for her earlier aloofness was gone. For the first time she and Marilyn were able to get genuinely acquainted with each other. To everyone's joy, they discovered that they liked each other.

Margarita's visit was an important turning point, the beginning of a highly treasured relationship between Marilyn and David's family. Shortly after the visit, Margarita sent Marilyn a lovely Bible with the inscription, "To Marilyn, our daughter Marilyn. Love, Mom and Dad."

Marilyn cried when she read those words. She knew then that everything was going to be all right. Today she says of David's parents, "Our relationship is marvelous. I couldn't ask for better in-laws."

David and Marilyn's first year in Colorado Springs was a special time of learning and growing. There were the normal adjustments to marriage, of course. They had assumed they knew all there was to know about each other, but they soon discovered that the real learning begins after a couple shares a life together.

Their interests quickly stretched beyond their home to include the First Baptist Church of Colorado Springs, where David and Marilyn were appointed sponsors of the single young adults. It was not a casual responsibility. The year 1968 brought with it numerous crises in the nation, touching the lives of young and old alike. But the young were especially vulnerable.

The Vietnam war was still raging. Strife was rampant on college campuses as young people joined protest marches, burned their draft cards, and rebelled against the Establishment. The drug problem was escalating as marijuana gained widespread acceptance among youth, and deadly LSD reached fad status. Families were breaking up. Some teenagers ran away from home to become hippies, more intent on "dropping out and turning on" than in becoming worthwhile citizens.

David and Marilyn found a microcosm of society's problems in their work with the young people. Several hippies in the group attempted to introduce liberal programs into the church. They set up coffee houses where dances were held and liquor was served—all in the name of Christianity. Often motorcycle gangs attended church only to disrupt the services. Their philosophy was, "We protest in the streets and get away with it, so why not in the church as well?"

David took a strong stand against such behavior. He even brought several aberrant young people under examination by the pastor, warning them that they would be physically removed from the church if they continued to misbehave.

There were other major issues that David and Marilyn felt compelled to confront. They wrote a letter of reprimand to the local council of churches for supporting the divisive activities of many radical young people. David also protested a radio program sponsored by the council of churches, because of its startlingly liberal stand on premarital sex and the use of drugs for "spiritual upliftment." David participated in a number of church symposiums aimed at shedding light on the problem of premarital sex, and he spoke frequently to single young adult groups at both his church and the local Presbyterian church. Throughout his two years in Colorado, David took a vigorous stand on numerous issues in his effort to help stem the tide of erosion within the church and, ultimately, within society itself.

But at times he felt extremely frustrated. "I'm fighting a losing battle," he would lament to Marilyn. "It seems that for every step I take forward, we fall two steps back."

"It's all right," Marilyn would reassure him. "You're doing a great job." During these days she had become the stable force in his life, the one who was quietly behind him, supporting him with her encouragement and prayers. "You've planted the seed, David. Others will water it, and someday the fruit will grow."

With new optimism in his voice, David would tell her appreciatively, "Honey, I get my strength from the Lord through your prayers."

Essentially David and Marilyn considered their two years in Colorado Springs a memorable experience—an exciting time of loving each other; of learning to cope, take stands, serve the Lord in a capacity of advising and guiding young people, and be responsible within the church structure.

They maintained an open door policy in their home. Young people could stop by at any time to have a bite to eat, play religious records, or just come and share their problems. David and Marilyn encouraged youths with special abilities to develop their talents, so that eventually several were singing on the local radio station, while others submitted their poems to religious magazines.

While stationed at the Fort Carson medical unit in Colorado Springs, David never saw a single GI. Because of his Ob/Gyn specialty, he treated only their dependents. He also did some consultation work for the Army. During his two-year stint, he was promoted from captain to major. He enjoyed his work, didn't feel pushed or pressured, and had regular eight-hour days, providing welcome leisure time to spend with his wife.

Sometimes the two of them took to the ski slopes at the Broadmoor Resort or spent an evening in town window-shopping (David's small military salary didn't allow for many purchases). On Sunday mornings before church, they ate out at a restaurant that offered breakfast for two for only two dollars.

While most of David and Marilyn's first two years of marriage was characterized by a spirit of love and harmony, one incident sparked a strong difference of opinion, precipitating their first major argument.

On a cold winter night in 1968, David and Marilyn lay in bed talking, comfortable and cozy while snow shrouded the world outside. They were discussing their favorite topic of conversation for the past several months—the impending birth of their first child. As they shared their hopes and dreams for their baby's future, one remark led to another, until they found themselves arguing over where their child would attend college.

"I think our purposes would be best served by sending our boy to a Christian college," said David solemnly. He was lying with his arms folded behind his neck, gazing through the darkness at the ceiling.

"Well, I don't see anything wrong with the public school system," said Marilyn. "It was good enough for me."

With ingratiating smugness, David launched into a thorough discourse on the advantages of a Christian education. Logically, meticulously, he outlined his reasons, step by step. As he spoke, his confidence grew. He sensed that he was nailing Marilyn to the wall with his arguments. The more he pontificated, the more pompous his tone became. Although he kept his eyes focused on the ceiling, he could feel Marilyn's irritation growing. Then just as he was congratulating himself on winning this round, he felt a sledgehammer fist slam into his stomach. In one agonizing instant the wind exploded from his lungs. The baleful noise resounded in the room as he doubled over in excruciating pain. Clutching his abdomen, he gasped for air. "W-What happened?" he croaked.

Immediately Marilyn jumped out of bed, turned on the light, and scrambled over to David, her face ghostly pale. "I'm sorry, David," she stammered. "I didn't mean . . . it just happened—"

He stared up at her in wounded astonishment. "Why—?"

Marilyn was nearly in tears now. "I don't know, David. It's . . . it's your way of arguing. You were so obnoxious. Even in the dark I could see your smile—just from the tone of your voice. You sounded so cocky and self-assured . . . I just lost control." Her voice broke with remorse. "I didn't even stop to think what I was doing. You—you are all right, aren't you?"

Gingerly David moved his torso. "That was a low blow, Babe," he rasped, "but I guess you didn't do any permanent damage."

"Aren't you furious with me?" asked Marilyn contritely, sitting down beside him.

David shook his head dazedly. "I'm too stunned to be angry."

"I had a sudden vision of you sending me home to California. I wondered how I'd ever explain this to my mother."

David chuckled, a baffled, spontaneous sound. "This can't be real. Our first fight . . . over where we're sending our son to college!" His arm circled her shoulder. "I think I'm OK, hon. How about you?"

"I felt terrific right after I hit you," she admitted. "But then I was scared out of my wits that I'd hurt you and that you'd send me away."

"I was scared too," he confessed. After a moment he began to laugh. "Do you realize the absolute silliness of this whole thing?" He patted her tummy. "Our baby has a while yet to decide about college—agreed?"

They both laughed with enormous relief as the tension between them dissipated. "This reminds me of a situation involving my folks," remarked David at last. "Before I was born they bought me a splendid piano. I guess they expected me to be a great piano virtuoso. But by the time I was old enough to play, the piano was infested with rats."

"Oh, David, no!"

"And the way my parents must have felt when they realized what they had done . . . that's just about how foolish I feel now."

TWENTY-TWO

Early in September 1969, three days before David was scheduled for discharge from the military, an incident occurred which could easily have spelled disaster for his little family. They were indeed a family now, since the birth of their son Mark David seven months before. What's more, Marilyn had unknowingly just become pregnant with their second child.

On this particular day, she and David were busily packing and cleaning house in preparation for their return to California. Around noon, David sent Marilyn out to get some Arby's roast beef sandwiches for lunch. She climbed into the VW, strapped Mark in his infant seat beside her, and drove off. David continued to clean the house, energetically scrubbing the walls and windows. He expected Marilyn to return in twenty or thirty minutes.

An hour passed, and David was growing increasingly concerned. Where was Marilyn? Why hadn't she returned? He telephoned the police and highway patrol; they had no report of an accident. He was reluctant to leave the house to look for her. What if she called and he wasn't there? But after another half hour had passed, he jumped into his car and sped over to Arby's to see if Marilyn was there. No sign of her VW. He checked inside. "No, the lady you describe hasn't been here," said the man behind the counter.

David dashed home and continued to wait in the silent house for some word of his wife and child. He paced the floor, stared anxiously out the window, and listened for the phone. He tried to pray, but his thoughts were fragmented, scattering before he could gather them into a rational statement. By now, more than two hours had passed. It was as if Marilyn and Mark had disappeared off the face of the earth.

Then, finally, the telephone rang. David answered, breathless. A toneless voice on the other end of the line said, "Dr. Hernandez, this is the emergency room at the base. We just brought in your wife and baby."

That noon, when Marilyn left for Arby's, she was feeling fine. She was tired, of course, but that was natural. There was so much to do to get ready to move. And she was hungry too. She hadn't eaten for several hours. Already she could imagine the luscious aroma of Arby's roast beef, thinly sliced and smothered in sauce.

But then, somehow she found herself, not at Arby's, but walking around inside a Safeway store. How did she get here? She meandered up and down the aisles, wondering what she had intended to purchase. Her mind was a blank. In frustration she picked up a box of teething cookies and headed for the checkout stand. But when she tried to pay for her purchase, she had trouble with the checker. He didn't seem to understand what she was saying. He eyed her suspiciously as she grew more and more flustered. People stared curiously. What was wrong with everyone? she wondered.

As she drove away from Safeway's, Marilyn's mind played cruel little tricks, ripping baffling holes in her memory. Where was she going? She was in the car, driving somewhere. Puzzled, she helped herself to some of the teething cookies. *Eat something, yes, a good idea.* She reached for another cookie. Markie babbled softly beside her, reaching out awkwardly for her shoulder. At moments he seemed startlingly close to her; then he seemed to recede. Everything appeared to pull back away from her, as if the world were out of reach. Where was she going? Where had she been? And how, in the name of Heaven, could she get back?

She was driving. Yes, hang on to that. She held the steering wheel in her hands, a firm grip. The road stretched out predictably—a straight gray highway, punctuated by telephone poles and drab, fleeting buildings. She forced her eyes to remain on the center white line. It was a guide, a marker, offering bleak security. *Stay to the right of the white line*, she told herself sternly. But why were so many drivers honking as they passed by?

Where am I going? she wondered again.

The holes in her memory were expanding, gaping outrageously. They kept her from forming comprehensible thoughts. The words refused to link; they spurned one another, faltered, dissolved. She began to feel waves of nausea attacking. Her skin felt cold, clammy, her hands wet on the steering wheel. Somewhere from the abyss of confusion in her brain sprang an impression, blurred, flimsy, but yes, a specific impression. *I am in trouble. In trouble!*

How long had she been driving? Was she actually still driving, or did she only imagine herself behind the wheel? Where was she? On a stretch of highway somewhere, but where?

She pulled over with an awkward jolt and stopped the car. She gazed vaguely at the automobiles whizzing by. Rolling down the window, she put her hand out and waved dreamily, automatically, watching herself from across a great chasm, feeling disconnected from both her mind and body.

After a while, she became aware of a voice, a man's voice, strange, urgent. "What's your name?" he insisted, staring through the window. "Are you on drugs? What did you take?"

She tried to reply, to snatch the words from their peculiar limbo in her mind and deliver them to her tongue. "I—I'm diabetic," she managed in a small, weak voice.

"Put her and the child in one of the vehicles," the stranger told a companion. "Take them to the base. Emergency!"

Later, as the confusion subsided, Marilyn overheard the doctor on the telephone. "Don't worry, Dr. Hernandez, your wife and baby are fine. Evidently your wife's blood sugar dropped significantly and she had a hypoglycemic reaction. She was totally disoriented when we found her. Lucky she happened to have some teething cookies to snack on, or it could have been worse. We found her in her car fifteen miles south of the base, on the highway to Canyon City. A convoy was coming back from maneuvers. The chaplain saw her wave and stopped to see what was wrong. He brought her in. We gave her glucose, and she's coming out of it now. In her condition she was sure lucky not to have an accident or get picked up by some weirdo. Sure lucky, I tell you!"

"Oh, it wasn't luck," said David, trembling slightly from tension and relief. "Thank God, we weren't depending on luck!"

In the following days, David and Marilyn praised God often for protecting her and Mark on that frightening day. David also wrote a letter of commendation to the chaplain for his inestimable act of service to the Hernandez family.

On September 8, 1969, David was released from the service. It had not been easy for him and Marilyn to decide where they should go from there. Several prestigious opportunities had been available. He had received an invitation to take a practice north of Sacramento, and to teach part-time at the medical school at the University of California at Davis. The offer looked good, but David and Marilyn didn't feel compelled to accept it.

David was also invited to join Dr. Seymour Polk in an impressive Ob/Gyn practice in Los Gatos, in the Santa Clara Valley. This offer appealed to him, for he would be close to his parents again for the first time since high school. And he would be able to affiliate himself with Stanford University, which had an extension at the Santa Clara County Medical Center.

But after prayerful consideration, David decided to return to White Memorial Medical Center in Los Angeles. He accepted an invitation to be chairman of the Department of Community Medicine and to join the teaching staff for the Department of Ob/Gyn. He would also serve as co-director of the Family Planning Clinic. In addition, he was given the option of becoming a faculty member in the school of medicine at the University of Southern California. He would receive a dual faculty appointment—to the Department of Ob/Gyn and to the Department of Community Medicine and Public Health.

David liked the idea of combining private practice with part-time teaching. And Marilyn was pleased at the prospect of being near her parents once more. So they both agreed: Southern California, here we come!

David, Marilyn, and Mark moved into a pleasant two-bedroom house only two blocks from her parents' home in San Gabriel. They were happy to be settled again in California. Marilyn enjoyed being a full-time wife and mother, and David found his new work both satisfying and challenging.

There was one incident during 1969 that cast a pall over David's joy. His good friend and former classmate Dr. Oral Fisher died of bone cancer. Just two years before, Oral had sung at David and Marilyn's wedding. A skilled ophthalmologist, he had been a brilliant yet humble man with a strong faith and extraordinary promise.

During the funeral service, David found himself feeling disconcerted and, frankly, a little bitter. His close friend was gone—and what a travesty of justice it seemed to be. But David couldn't ignore Oral's exemplary testimony. He knew that Oral had maintained a close walk with Christ. Then a startling thought struck David: How tragic if one never discovers the privilege of fellowship with the Lord until he is pressed by the hard edge of death!

I, too, must lock into Jesus more firmly, he resolved. *God is our only fortress. Otherwise, our lives are unfortified cities.*

But in a few days other concerns took priority in David's mind. His sense of urgency for spiritual renewal faded. It would be nearly five years before he would follow through on his resolution to "lock into Jesus more firmly."

In the meantime, David and Marilyn's second child, Michael Laurence, was born on May 18, 1970. This birth, like the first, was performed by cesarean section. With two adorable children, a lovely home, prestige, and financial security, David and Marilyn felt that their life was very nearly perfect. They even built a swimming pool in the backyard—a sure sign of the good life in balmy Southern California. But toward the end of the summer they caught a stark, frightening glimpse of the tenuousness of human security and temporal provisions.

It happened one afternoon while they were enjoying a family get-together around the pool with Marilyn's parents, her sister Charlene, and Charlene's nine-year-old son Jeff. Nineteen-month-old Mark was sitting on the steps of the pool playing with a rubber boat while Jeff swam happily in the deep end.

David and Marilyn were saying good-bye to her mother when they heard Jeff scream, "Mark! Mark!"

David whirled around and spotted his son in the middle of the pool, rolling and turning, his arms flailing the air, his head bobbing momentarily on the surface of the water, then disappearing from view.

"He's drowning!" cried Marilyn, panic-stricken.

David dove into the water, gathered the boy into his arms, and returned to the side of the pool. Immediately he compressed Mark's lungs to expel the water. The youngster coughed and sputtered, but he was okay.

"Oh, David, it happened so fast," Marilyn cried, cuddling her son and kissing his chubby, tear-stained cheeks. "We were just seconds from disaster—that's what's so frightening!"

David reached out and tousled Mark's wet hair, then drew the boy to him. "You know, Marilyn, as parents we're so vulnerable," he said weakly. "There's no way we can protect our children from every risk. They will suffer hurts, and so will we. We can only try to minimize the risks."

Eventually the vivid terror of that moment faded as David and Marilyn became absorbed in more practical, mundane matters. With two children in the home, the Hernandez house seemed to be shrinking before their eyes. Inevitably they had to find a larger place. While looking around in the San Marino area, they found a beautiful, captivating home which they both loved instantly. On impulse they made an offer. Although the amount was significantly lower than the asking price, it was much more than David and Marilyn had anticipated spending on a house.

"Don't count on this one, Babe," he warned her gently. "It's not likely that the owners will accept our offer. Even if they did, I probably couldn't get the financing."

As it turned out, the owners did accept their offer and the finance company approved the loan. Suddenly David and Marilyn faced the prospect of having to come up with 30,000 dollars within ninety days.

"Thirty thousand dollars?" cried Marilyn, horrified. "David, we don't have that kind of money."

David's expression reflected the despair in his wife's voice. "I know, hon. We blew it this time. We jumped into this thing without even praying or seeking the Lord's guidance."

"What can we do now?"

"We can't break the deal or we'll lose the money we've already put down," said David miserably. "Let's start making things right by getting on our knees and asking God to forgive us for being so impetuous."

Over the next several days David and Marilyn juggled their budget, desperate to find a solution to their dilemma.

"We can probably clear 10,000 on our present home," said David.

"Great," returned Marilyn. "That leaves just 20,000 dollars."

"All right. We'll budget every penny. I'll even 'brown bag' it to the hospital."

Marilyn began to catch his spirit of enthusiasm. "OK. We'll live on beans. No credit cards, no purchases. We won't go anywhere except to church—and the grocery store."

"For more beans."

"Right. Lots of beans!"

"It won't be easy," cautioned David.

"I know. But we'll do it. We'll get the money."

True to their resolves, at the end of three months, they made the down payment. They had scrimped, cut their spending to the bone, and were ultimately forced to use all their savings; but they met their commitment. The home, where they still live today, turned out to be the best financial investment of their lives.

"It was a trying experience," David reflected later, "but we learned . . . we grew. The Lord not only forgave us, he made up our deficit, even though we sought him after the fact."

Over the next three years, the texture and pattern of living for the Hernandez family was rich, warm, and variegated. Their lives were full and rewarding. David and Marilyn delighted in their healthy, growing boys. David's medical career flourished. He was financially secure, with sufficient insurance coverage, savings, and a nice investment portfolio. Young and energetic, he was convinced that the "good life" was upon him. He felt insulated from harm.

However, he still had not established the firm relationship with God he had intended. His fellowship with Christ was admittedly sporadic. But there was time to work on that . . . tomorrow.

In 1973, David faced a major, unprecedented crossroad in his career. He was offered a prestigious position as an associate medical director with the Los Angeles County Hospital and the USC Medical School, with an annual salary of 60,000 dollars. It was a rare, highly attractive proposal.

David prayed seriously about the matter, discussed it thoroughly with Marilyn, and sought the counsel of his good friends, Dr. James Dobson and Dr. Victor Herlacher. But it wasn't until he read Psalm 119 in *The Living Bible* that God spoke to him in a clear, consummate voice:

I told you my plans . . . Now give me your instructions. . . . Lord, don't let me make a mess of things. . . . Just tell me what to do and I will do it, Lord. As long as I live I'll wholeheartedly obey. . . . Help me to prefer obedience to making money! Turn me away from wanting any other plan than yours. Revive my heart toward you. Reassure me that your promises are for me, for I trust and revere you.

After reading those words, David knew what decision he had to make. He refused the impressive offer and remained in private practice and teaching. It was the right choice. God's peace swept over him.

Later that year David was invited to share his testimony with the congregation of his church, the First Church of the Nazarene in Pasadena. He stood up and spoke with the quiet authority of a man who had every facet of his life superbly under control. After talking at some length about his family background and personal experiences, David concluded, "If I had any pearls of wisdom to leave with you, they would be: First, learn to live perceptively, seeing everything in view of eternity. Trust in *him!* Second, remember, you have not chosen God; he has chosen you. Third, know and understand yourself. Find integration and salvation in Christ. He will grant you a sense of destiny as you meet your daily tasks.

"Finally," he said, his gaze moving slowly, entreatingly over the congregation, "the world does not so much need men of great intellect as of noble and regenerated character and ambition. It needs men in whom ability is controlled by steadfast principle."

As David shared that day how God had blessed and instructed him, he had no idea how soon he would be called upon to exhaust all his spiritual reserves for the most formidable and crushing battle of his life.

TWENTY-THREE

What does a strong, happy, seemingly invincible man do when he has been handed a death sentence? That was the staggering question that confronted David and his family in 1974.

It began in January when David felt unusually fatigued. His stamina was slipping; his mind often succumbed to an oppressive weariness.

"You're working too hard," Marilyn chided from time to time.

"I know," David admitted. "But I have responsibilities."

"Can't you slow down . . . cut something out?"

"What do you suggest, Babe? My private practice? My classes at White Memorial and USC?"

"But you schedule so many patients, sometimes more than you can handle."

"Hon, that's just the way it is. Besides, you know many of my patients are Mexican-Americans who speak little or no English. They wouldn't feel at ease with an Anglo doctor. You don't expect me to turn them away, do you?"

"No," she conceded. "But then how about eliminating a few committees and community programs?"

"I have people depending on me there too, sweetheart. It's important for me to be on the admissions committee and minority screening committee at USC. And I can't turn down opportunities to lecture on family-oriented issues, especially when they involve the Spanish community."

"But, David, you can't take on the needs of the whole world, or even of your own people," argued Marilyn. "Your family depends on you too. We deserve some of your time. You've been working twelve . . . sixteen . . . sometimes eighteen-hour days."

"I can manage, hon."

"Then why are you so tired all the time? You should have a checkup, David. How long has it been?"

"Are your serious?" he scoffed. "I'm perfectly healthy, have been all my life. I'm quite capable of enduring long, strenuous hours of work."

"You think you can do anything," she gibed.

"I can . . . anything I set my mind to," he answered with a teasing smile.

Throughout February David's schedule remained cluttered, if not crammed. In March he began to experience nausea thirty to forty minutes after meals.

"What's wrong?" Marilyn asked with concern after dinner one evening.

Ashen-faced, David met her gaze. "I don't know, hon. It might be pylorospasm from stress." He paused, rubbing his abdomen. "Or possibly gastritis from hyperacidity."

"OK, doctor," she said gently, "what you're saying is that you feel sick to your stomach."

He nodded, in obvious discomfort. "One thing's certain," he added in a weak attempt at humor, "I can't blame it on your good cooking!"

"Well, this isn't the first time you've felt sick, David. I'm going to call a specialist tomorrow."

Over the next two months David underwent extensive testing, including blood tests and X-rays which revealed dysfunction of both the gallbladder and the liver.

"It can't be serious, can it?" David questioned his colleagues. "I have no pain, no fever, no jaundice."

His physicians were equally puzzled by the findings. "We can't be sure whether two concomitant diseases exist," said one internist.

"Or whether it's a singular disease with secondary effects," said the other consultant.

Later, when surgeons were consulted, they opted for chronic gallbladder disease. Because of the confused medical picture, David was urged to repeat the liver profile tests every two weeks. He did so, and the first two or three times the battery of tests indicated an improvement. With these encouraging results, David and Marilyn rejoiced, praying fervently that surgery could still be averted. "If not," said David wryly, "I'm already reconciled to parting with my gallbladder, even if it means giving up Mexican food."

But subsequent tests revealed an ominous reversing trend. By May it was clear that exploratory surgery was inevitable.

"How can I have an operation now?" David asked Marilyn one evening as they sat together on the sofa before the fireplace. It was a rhetorical question. They both knew he would have to undergo surgery, the sooner the better.

David stood up and placed one hand on the mantle in a deliberate, ruminative gesture. He looked at Marilyn. "All my June and July elective surgeries are pending." When Marilyn made no reply, he continued with persuasive urgency. "Babe, you know how it is in my line of work. Mothers often put off surgery until the children are home for the summer and fathers can take vacation time to help out. I'm booked solid."

"Well, you'll have to figure out something, David. You've got to take care of your own health."

Realizing the truth of Marilyn's words, David launched an intensive program to clear his backlog of surgeries. Through May, June, and July he performed from one to three surgeries a day, until his calender was clear. His own operation was scheduled for July 23, 1974.

Two weeks before his surgery, David received some pleasant, momentarily distracting news. His name had been selected for inclusion in the book, *Who's Who in the State of California*. He felt extremely honored and pleased.

That same week a curious incident occurred which would take on profound significance for David in the days ahead. He was in the backyard watering Marilyn's garden when the phone rang. He put down the hose and rushed inside, then returned minutes later to an astonishing sight. The fig tree, with its huge V-shaped trunk, lay on its side, uprooted.

David looked around, incredulous. The tree had been standing only minutes ago—strong, sturdy, loaded with fruit. There was no wind; there had been no earthquake. He hadn't even heard a noise. Yet without warning, without apparent reason, the tree had fallen.

David scratched his head in bewilderment and murmured, "This can't happen. It must be a trick." He looked around dubiously. "I'm not on 'Candid Camera,' am I?" he said, only half in jest.

He noticed that the tree's major root system showed fungus in the soil, but there had been no external evidence of decadence or disease. David shook his head slowly and walked back toward the house. "I'll chop it up for firewood on Saturday," he told himself.

On Thursday, David's Uncle Vincent stopped by for a brief visit. David showed him the tree, adding offhandedly, "I sure hated losing it like that."

"David, do you want this tree?" asked his uncle.

Surprise registered on David's face. "Yes, of course. But how—?"

"Then get me three long two-by-fours, a hammer, wire, nails, and a shovel."

After David had brought the necessary tools, his uncle stooped down and pointed toward the ground where the fig tree had been. "See this, David? This tree has contracted fungus. It has a watering trough that it doesn't need. What it requires is more soil packed up against the trunk. And look here. You've surrounded it with too much fertilizer. The soil is too rich and the ground isn't firm enough."

David nodded, unconvinced.

Uncle Vincent stood up, still speaking. "The roots must grow deep and out to have strength. I think if we pick it up and put it back, it might survive. One of the two trunks still has rootage attached."

David figured he might as well humor his uncle. After all, he didn't want to offend the man, and he could always chop up the dead tree later. Together they lifted the fig tree into place, packed soil hard against its trunk, and supported it with the three beams. Aloud, for his uncle's sake, David jovially wished the tree well, but in his mind he had already marked it hopeless. He couldn't guess that in the uncertain weeks ahead, that fig tree would hold a prominent place in his troubled thoughts about his own life.

On Monday, July 22, 1974, David made his usual hospital rounds, discharged his patients from the preceding week's surgeries, and that afternoon entered the hospital as a patient. His parents flew in from San Jose and joined Marilyn at his bedside that evening. David was cheerful, even laughing and making jokes.

"I'm sure it's nothing serious," he told his mother reassuringly. "I'm just having what they call an exploratory procedure. I imagine they will do a simple cholecys-tectomy—removal of the gallbladder. You know what that means, Mom," he added with a wink, "I'll have to cut out the tortillas and enchiladas and hot peppers."

"I'll thank God if that's all you have to cut out," replied Margarita.

"We're convinced it's nothing serious," repeated Marilyn with forced lightness.

Before going home, the family prayed with David. Each one held on to that meaningful phrase, *nothing serious*.

Later that evening, David and Marilyn's close friends Steve and Doris Reed paid him a visit. Alluding to Steve's occupation in law, David jested, "It's amazing how lawyers always show up preoperatively in case one wishes to make proper legal arrangements!" Everyone laughed; it was funny, a joke. It meant nothing.

Early the next morning, on Tuesday, July 23, Marilyn and David's parents arrived at the hospital and prayed with him before he was taken to surgery. Marilyn, Margarita, and Jose spent the next three and one-half hours in the waiting room, sitting idly, saying little, sometimes drinking coffee or pacing the floor. The minutes crept by.

Finally several doctors approached, their expressions grim. One, a close friend of David's, had tears in his eyes. Dr. Vannix, the surgeon, still in his greens, approached and looked gravely at Marilyn.

Jose put his arm protectively around Margarita and whispered, "Hold on, honey. I've got a feeling there's bad news."

"How is he?" Marilyn asked quickly.

"It's not good."

As if an actual chill had descended on the room, Marilyn shivered involuntarily. "Tell us—" she murmured.

The doctor's voice was husky. "His liver is severely damaged," he said slowly. "We found a mass of scar tissue at the base of the common bile duct—the main drainage tube from the liver." When Marilyn remained silent, he continued. "We removed numerous lymph nodes from the surrounding area. The frozen section was benign, but it will be three or four days before we get the final pathology report."

"So there's no cancer?" queried Marilyn.

"So far. We biopsied the liver and opened and inspected the gallbladder. It was remarkably normal."

"Then what's wrong with David?" she questioned.

Dr. Vannix cleared his throat; his tone deepened. "We've tentatively diagnosed a disease called sclerosing cholangitis."

"I—I've never heard of it," said Marilyn haltingly.

"No, not many have. It's a rare disease of unknown origin—a scarring of the biliary tree."

"How . . . how serious is it?"

There was a pause, then: "Extremely."

Marilyn glanced at David's parents. They looked back at her. "I don't know if I'm hearing you right—" Marilyn began, her voice sounding slightly strangled.

"Is my son going to be all right?" interrupted Jose.

The doctor's face was expressionless, a mask. "I don't know."

"What do you mean?" demanded Jose.

"In cases like this—and admittedly our experience is limited—the prognosis is poor."

"Poor? How poor, doctor?" Jose persisted.

"The survival rate is profoundly limited."

They stared at him, stunned. Marilyn felt her mind reeling uncontrollably. "Are you telling us . . . you're not saying he has only a—a few years to live?"

The surgeon's gaze dropped momentarily. Into the gaping vacuum of silence he inserted the words, "I am so sorry." The words hung in the air, stark, lethal, immobilizing.

TWENTY-FOUR

When Marilyn, Margarita, and Jose finally saw David, he was back in his own room and just beginning to open his eyes. Groggily he mumbled, "I want to see Dr. Vannix."

Jose summoned David's surgeon, who visited briefly, then told Marilyn, "I'll be back in the morning to talk to David about his condition. He'll be more alert then."

The next morning Marilyn arrived early at the hospital and was at David's bedside when he awoke.

"Hi, sweetheart," he murmured, giving her a wan smile.

She took his hand, then leaned over and kissed him. "Hi, honey."

"Was—was there any cancer?" he asked.

"No, David, but—"

Before she could continue, Dr. Vannix arrived on morning rounds. She greeted him with a mixture of anxiety and relief. He pulled a chair over beside David's bed and sat down. His expression was solemn as he told David what he had already told the family. Vannix went on to explain, "The common bile duct was essentially blocked, David. We were faced with the dilemma of decompressing the liver. The saving grace was your normal gallbladder. We used it to shunt the obstruction to the jejunum."

"But the prognosis," said David weakly, "it doesn't sound good."

"We can't be sure. We know so little about the pathophysiology of the disease."

David's face contorted slightly. "I want the truth. How long can I expect?"

Dr. Vannix's brow furrowed. "I can't tell you how long, David. No one knows the progression of this disease. But," he admitted reluctantly, "it could mean a very shortened life expectancy."

The physician's words struck with cataclysmic force. David began to sob.

That evening Pastor Earl Lee visited David. The two men exchanged casual bits of conversation. The minister was warm and encouraging, David polite but subdued. "I chose my surgeon wisely," said David, "and the rest is up to God."

Pastor Lee nodded. He met David's gaze. Without warning, David's tears came again, shatteringly. He groaned, "My whole life is fragmenting . . . dismantling before my eyes. I feel abandoned by God, marooned on an island, shipwrecked."

Pastor Lee could offer only meager consolation. Together, he and David bowed their heads and pleaded for God's mercy.

For David, the long nightmare was just beginning. He found himself facing sleepless nights, plagued by the questions, *Why me? Why our family? Why would a loving God permit this?* He thought of his two little boys growing up without a father and his wife struggling alone. He was assaulted by vivid images of Michael and Mark reaching for their mother's hand, saying, "Don't cry, Mommy. We will take care of you."

When he did sleep, he suffered strange, terrifying dreams in which he would awaken in a grave, helpless and unable to participate or rejoice with the living. It was as if his childhood nightmares and fears of death had reared up hideously to devour him, to crush his desperate grip on sanity. .

He became entrenched in self-pity. He called it an "honest quandary," but it opened the door to bitterness and resentment. He tried to explain his suffering in rational terms, but he could find no plausible answer.

Whenever Marilyn visited David in the hospital, they prayed and cried together and turned to the Scriptures. David told her of his inner struggles. "I plead for God to make faith rational and meaningful," he said. "I want a dividend, a share in faith. But I don't know how to enter into that experience."

"But you've spent your life in Sunday school and church. You've studied about faith. Surely—"

"That's just it. I'm trapped between theory and practice. I keep running into cul-de-sacs, dead-end streets. I know real faith doesn't come from philosophizing about it. But faith eludes me. Instead, I'm bombarded by questions. I hear the words, *I'm doomed and I can't do a thing about it!* And I wonder, Why would God allow my strength and capacity to be reduced, maybe even snuffed out, at the prime of my life and career? How much can I take? How much will our family have to suffer?" He reached for her hand and clasped it urgently. "I don't want to feel this way, Marilyn. I don't want to be trapped by bitter feelings."

"You won't be, David. We're coming through this. Our pastor, our church, our family and friends are surrounding us with their love and prayers."

"I know," said David, glancing around the room. "Look at all the plants and flowers and cards I've received." He managed a weak smile. "Jim Dobson telephoned and said, 'Dave, we are standing around you like a wall, in prayer.'"

On Saturday, David's fourth post-op day, his parents prepared to return to the Bay area. On their last visit to the hospital, Jose prayed in Spanish for his son. Large, warm tears landed on David's arm as his father leaned over the rail, clutching his son's hand and pleading with God. Jose said, "Almighty God, we present to you our son, our only son. We love him so very much. We don't understand why he has to suffer with this affliction." As Jose continued to pray, the truth dawned on him and he exclaimed, "Neither do we understand why you would give your only beloved Son to die and redeem humanity." At that moment, David sensed in his father an agonizing transition into peace and understanding.

Just before David was dismissed from the hospital, he

asked Dr. Vannix to lend him the medical literature on his illness. Later the surgeon reluctantly gave Marilyn the material, with the comment, "I knew David would have his secretary research it if I didn't oblige, so I decided to save her the trouble."

At home, surrounded by his family and familiar things, David's spirits began to improve. He took pleasure in Marilyn's attentiveness and concern. He felt himself settling into a state of near-complacency. The numbness was almost pleasant compared with his earlier anger and frustration. He walked often in the garden and took particular satisfaction in observing the progress of his fig tree. His uncle had been right. One trunk of the V-shaped tree was actually surviving.

During his convalescence he tried not to think much about his illness. When it did enter his mind, he told himself it couldn't be as bad as he had originally been led to believe. Regardless, he knew as a doctor that he ought to become more acquainted with the nature of his condition. So one day he asked Marilyn for the literature the doctor had given him.

"It's downstairs in the den," she replied. "I'll get it later."

The next day he asked her again. She said, "Your sister Dee has been reading it. I'll check with her after a while."

By the third day, David said impatiently, "Look, sweetheart, let me have the material." Marilyn got it and handed it to him without a word.

As David studied the literature on sclerosing cholangitis, he understood Marilyn's hesitancy. An article from the April 1973 *American Surgeon* stated, "Many patients' conditions run a fulminating course ending in death by liver failure, bleeding esophageal varices, biliary cirrhosis or biliary sepsis." Another article from the June 1971 issue of *The American Journal of Surgery* presented the opinions of several doctors regarding the prognosis of the disease. One physician asserted that "survival does not exceed two to three years despite all measures." Another doctor predicted "an average of six years of life from onset of symptoms." Some opinions were more optimistic, but David's mind had already seized upon the essential message of the material. It was there in black and white: A rare, unpredictable illness had commandeered his body; it carried with it a death sentence.

With staggering clarity David realized he had not accepted this truth. Somehow he had circumvented the facts; he had clung to the bleak, anesthetizing comfort of complacency and self-imposed ignorance.

Now the truth rocketed into his consciousness with a paroxysm of anguish, tearing painfully into his deepest being. He looked at Marilyn with tears of desolation. They embraced and wept in each other's arms. For a long time they sat together, bound by love and grief, praying. Finally David began to talk. He had to verbalize what he was feeling now.

"I always considered the truth sweet and soothing . . . calming . . . composing," he said, choosing his words with a controlled articulation. But his voice suddenly broke with emotion as he said, "I have never known the truth to be so painful! It's so ironic, Marilyn. All my medical expertise can't save me. My colleagues and my connections with the academic world can't change the prognosis."

He continued speaking with a deep, compelling urgency, his words spilling over one another. "Skilled surgeons can't alter the situation. My life insurance policies can't give me an extension on life. My financial investments can't grant me a reprieve. My professionalism, my prestige, nothing, absolutely nothing can salvage my life." He paused and breathed deeply, as if absorbing the grim meaning of his own words.

Then he gazed at Marilyn with a mournful intensity. "I am completely at the mercy of Almighty God. I am stripped of all my securities. Oh, hon, the truth is painful. It stings!"

Gently Marilyn, fighting back her own tears, murmured, "But God's Word says the truth shall set us free. We have to hold on to that, David. We have to pull ourselves out of this."

David shook his head doubtfully. "A person can rise from under the rubble if restoration is within reach. He can surface from the quicksand when mental and physical stamina is intact . . . when strength and vitality are not crippled.''

"But would you choose to depend on your own strength if you did have it?" asked Marilyn quietly.

"I know what you're saying," David replied. "Our only real strength is in Christ. He alone is the truth that frees us. Intellectually I know these things, but how do I live them? How do I draw upon his strength to cope with what I'm facing now?''

"You can't . . . only *he* can," said Marilyn, her voice quavering slightly. "But, David, I honestly believe he can and will sustain you.''

David stared somberly into space. "I feel utterly helpless, Marilyn. All the props have been knocked out from under me. I can only say, I want to believe; God help my unbelief.''

"That's a beginning," said Marilyn.

A few days later, while David took his customary walk in the garden, he stopped by the fig tree. The tree had become a familiar friend. It was almost as if David and the tree had something in common, as if they shared some sort of obscure bond. He chided himself for the silly notion.

Then, incredibly, an insight struck him with staggering force. *He and the tree were extraordinarily alike!* God in his boundless grace had given David a living parable.

"That's it, isn't it, Lord?" he said aloud. "You are showing me myself in this tree. I too was once strong, robust, healthy, and productive. But my rootage was shallow and infested with fungus. The comforts and conveniences of life . . . the accumulation of things . . . royal treatment of overwatering . . . too much fertilizer.''

He reached out instinctively and rubbed the tree's rough bark. "I had position, prestige, influence, and money," he continued plausibly. "I thought those things would keep me vibrant and healthy, but the tree fell. It didn't even require a breeze to topple it." He gazed up at the branches, the rich green leaves, the bountiful fruit. "It was I who fell, Lord," he confessed. "I was ready to be cast out, to be chopped into firewood. But, Father, you are there, even now—I sense it—picking me up, supporting me. Oh, God, pack the soil of your Word around this broken trunk. Buttress me with your presence. I pray that by your grace the fruit on the remaining trunk will be acceptable."

Those hours in the garden, praying, renewing his relationship with God, learning the lesson of the fig tree, were vital for David. Christ himself became David's bridge from despair to trust. In the days that followed, as David diligently studied the Scriptures, he felt the roots of his faith growing deeper. Daily he struggled with the hard lesson of patience—walking slowly, reordering his life-style, realigning priorities, pruning the dead trunk of his old nature. David had been a Christian for many years. But now, at last, he had kept his promise of five years before, at the death of his friend Oral Fisher, to firmly "lock in" to Christ, to establish a daily, vital walk with God.

TWENTY-FIVE

There was no miracle drug to heal David's body. His doctors instituted steroid therapy, also utilizing antibiotics to prevent a secondary bacterial infection. But there was little improvement in his condition. In fact, complications from the steroids caused a metabolic imbalance, producing chemical diabetes. So the treatment was abandoned.

Two months after surgery, David resumed his medical practice, although his activities were necessarily restricted. Adequate rest and proper nutrition were vital. Over the next two years he suffered intermittent setbacks which brought periods of discouragement. In a spirit of struggling optimism, he told friends, "I'm keeping my eyes on the Lord, not on my liver." But both David and Marilyn kept a prayer on their lips for the complete restoration of liver function. While maintaining a steadfast hope for David's physical wholeness, they sought to live the admonition of 1 Thessalonians 5:18: "In every thing give thanks: for this is the will of God in Christ Jesus concerning you."

In 1976 David underwent a thorough examination to reevaluate his condition. Tests revealed little, if any, improvement; but at least there was no worsening of the disease. For that he and Marilyn praised God.

The paradox of devastation at the peak of life—what David termed "noonday destruction"—propelled him into a wholehearted regimen of prayer and Bible study. He felt an increasing hunger to know God, to explore more fully, more deeply, the facets and potential of spiritual interchange. He discovered dimensions of fellowship with Christ that he hadn't imagined. Jesus was personal and absolutely trustworthy; he was infinitely loving—sharing David's tears, upholding him through the valley of the shadow of death.

In David's times of deepest distress, God became the perfect Communicator, a caring Heavenly Father accessible and involved in David's frailties. Through persistent prayer (and influenced by Erling and Marge Wold's book, *What Do I Have to Do—Break my Neck?*), David discovered an awesome principle for spiritual communion: *God bends to me as I bend to him.* David tagged this process "meaningful dialogue." As he implemented his new approach to prayer, three Scripture passages in the Gospel of John took on paramount importance (John 14:13, 14; 15:7; 16:23, 24). From these passages David derived a concept of the wholeness of prayer. Threading through each verse was the main theme of receiving whatever one asks for in Jesus' name; but three sub-themes were also evident:

that the Father may be glorified in the Son
and my words abide in you
that your joy may be full

For David, having incorporated these verses into his thinking, the process of "meaningful dialogue" with God went something like this:

He prayed, "God, I beg of you to perform the impossible. Heal me, please!"

God responded, "If this is the way in which the Father may be glorified in the Son. . . ."

Then David replied, "OK, God, if you want me to remain this way with my infirmities, then I accept it."

God's Word came back to him, "My will is that your joy may be full."

David's excitement mounted as he began to see and understand the principles and purpose of prayer. He was able to say, honestly, by faith, "I accept death, recovery, suffering, whatever, as long as you are with me!"

And God's reassurance came, "As you are abiding in me, so my words abide in you."

Eagerly David shared with Marilyn what the Lord was teaching him. "Honey, God's answers to life's dilemmas are often locked in mysteries which are unveiled to us only through persistent prayer. God is the perfect Communicator. He not only speaks, but he listens; he not only listens, but he speaks. And throughout this exchange is intertwined the theme, 'He cares . . . I care.'

"You see the idea, Marilyn? We don't try to manipulate God; we don't threaten or demand. We *dialogue.* We speak; then we listen while he speaks. We go back and forth, expressing our needs, allowing him to talk to us, teach us. Hon, what joy there is in such communion!"

"It sounds good, David," said Marilyn with a warm, supportive smile.

"I want to tell you something else too," he continued, staring reflectively at his hands. He had picked up a book and was turning it over absently. "I'm no longer asking God why."

"You mean about your illness?"

"Yes, hon. I've moved away from the *whys.* 'Why' is a word weighed down with bitterness, engendered with confrontation. It's a demand for an explanation. It insists on accountability. It doesn't lead to dialogue. But thank God, I'm past the *whys* with our Savior."

David put the book down and looked tenderly at Marilyn. "There's another area of my life that God has been speaking to me about," he said quietly. "For years I've played the part of the average American father, caught up in the work ethic, putting my profession above everything else. But I realize now that my family must take priority. Aside from God, nothing is more precious to me than my family. I love you and the boys with all my heart. I feel as if I can't get enough of being with you."

Marilyn came over and sat beside him, slipping into his arms. "We feel that way too, David. We need you so much."

One Thursday night a few weeks after their conversation,

David was scheduled to speak to the Victors Sunday School Class at his church. He left work early that afternoon so that he could finish preparing some materials at home for the seven P.M. session. But when he arrived home at three-thirty, he felt weak and feverish. As he showered, his weakness increased.

Within minutes he could hardly move. He crawled into bed and lay there, helpless. All his muscles ached, his breathing was rapid, and he experienced severe nausea and chills.

Marilyn, clearly distressed, gave him aspirin and applied cool compresses on his forehead. "Honey, it must be another bout of cholangitis. You can't go anywhere tonight like this," she said firmly. "Let me call Vic Herlacher and cancel the session."

"No," said David, just as firmly. "I'll sleep awhile. Wake me at five. I'll see how I feel then."

At six-thirty David struggled out of bed and dressed. Marilyn entered the bedroom just as he was adjusting his tie.

"What are you doing out of bed?" she cried.

"I have a meeting at seven."

"You belong in bed. I told you to let me reschedule the meeting."

"No," said David flatly. "I'm going."

"Then I'll drive you," said Marilyn. "Your sister Dee will watch the boys."

"Let's pray first," suggested David. They sat together on the bed. He prayed, "Dear God, I just ask for strength enough to deliver my talk tonight. Then I'll return immediately to bed."

Marilyn helped David down the stairs. He maneuvered himself slowly into the car, knowing any excess movement would precipitate severe nausea. He felt sweaty and clammy; his mind struggled for clarity of thought.

At nearly every intersection Marilyn glanced worriedly at David. "Want to go back?"

"I'm tempted," he admitted faintly. "There's no place I'd rather be than home in bed."

"I'll turn around," she offered.

"No, go on. I've come this far."

After what seemed an interminable drive, they arrived at the church and pulled into the parking lot. Entering the church, Marilyn carried the projector and slides in one hand and gave David the other arm for support.

While waiting to be introduced, David pleaded with the Lord for a clear mind and a facility with words. "And please don't let me collapse on the spot," he added silently, urgently.

Then he heard his name and sensed everyone's eyes turning his way. Automatically he walked to the podium and began to speak. Every word was an effort, forced out by sheer willpower. But David would not surrender to his weakness. *Keep them going,* he told himself sharply, *one word after another.*

Incredibly, five minutes into his presentation he sensed a powerful surge of strength. The energy flowed through his body, into his muscles and limbs. He felt himself speaking suddenly with release and freedom; he could hardly comprehend the dramatic sense of well-being that flooded his mind. He finished his presentation with confidence and ease.

On returning home that evening, David sat down to a full Mexican dinner. He ate eagerly and survived the burritos and hot sauce without a bit of nausea.

"I can't believe you're eating like this," exclaimed Marilyn, giving him a second helping of refried beans.

"I can't believe how good I feel," marveled David between bites.

"Well, the next time you have a bout of colangitis, we'll just set up a speaking engagement for you. It seems to do wonders."

The next morning David and Marilyn learned one significant reason for David's startling recovery. At sunrise their boys, Michael and Mark, bounded into the bedroom and jumped excitedly on the bed with a story to tell. Last evening Auntie Dee had gathered them together for a special time of intercessory prayer. The youngsters had prayed simply, earnestly, "Please, Jesus, make Daddy well . . . just now . . . right now." They had no doubt but that God had heard their prayer.

On Sunday morning, May 16, 1976, David shared with the congregation of his church what God was doing in his life. Toward the end of his message he said, "Many of you here today are walking wounded. You mask your fragmented spirit with a firm handshake and gallant step, or with a plastic smile and Revlon makeup. But inside you are shattered. You have lost the center, the matrix of your life. That hub, that most important thing, may be your marriage, your career, a loved one, or some possession. But in losing that cherished center of your life, you feel you have lost everything."

He paused. There was a poignant silence over the large audience. "I invite you to make Jesus Christ the eternal center of your life. He is always available, always satisfying. Life disappoints, disintegrates; Christ alone remains faithful."

Again he hesitated, allowing his words to take hold. "Many of us, by our actions, shrink from the miracle that would change our lives. We are safe and secure in our self-pity, accustomed to our burdens. My own search for the salvaging of a physical dilemma became a search for a relationship with God. I came before him starkly naked, stripped of all pretense, reduced to essentials, released from the trappings of theology. And I found a loving God willing to channel me into a profound wholeness, where healing is not an end in itself but merely a part of that total wholeness offered. I am ready, open for his complete healing . . . either here or in eternity. In the meantime, I will praise God and serve him and wait patiently."

TWENTY-SIX

David and Marilyn had tapped their deepest spiritual reserves to cope with David's illness; they had come to accept the fact that he lived in jeopardy. They took solace in the fact that at least Marilyn, in spite of her diabetes, was healthy and whole; she would always be there for the boys, even if David was not. But in 1977 even this assumption was shattered, as a major new crisis loomed to threaten Marilyn's life.

It began early in the year with a bout of flu. The bug spread through the family, afflicting the boys, then Marilyn, and finally David. David, Mark, and Michael quickly recovered, but Marilyn remained weak and incapacitated for several weeks. She also began to notice discomfort in her abdomen, radiating to the area of her right kidney. She coughed constantly and slept with a heating pad to ease the pain in her side. When the cough was especially harsh, she spent the night in the guest room so that David could rest undisturbed.

In March, when Marilyn's discomfort still persisted, David ordered a battery of twelve tests—a profile of her liver, lungs, heart, and kidneys. The results indicated that everything was normal. Marilyn visited her internist for her annual exam; again nothing unusual was found. But the nagging pain continued.

David grew increasingly concerned. Marilyn wasn't a hypochondriac or a complainer. Most of the time she was a jovial, happy-go-lucky person. Something had to be seriously wrong, but what?

Toward the last of April David ordered a barium enema, an upper G.I. examination, and gallbladder X-rays. When he told Marilyn, she moaned, "Oh, David, no. The biggest insult to mankind is a barium enema!"

Nevertheless, she underwent the tests the following week. Afterward, she felt drained and tired, but happy to have the ordeal over.

By mid-afternoon on Wednesday, David received a message to telephone Dr. Roberts in radiology at the Community Hospital of San Gabriel. David still had three patients in the waiting room, but he slipped aside to make the call. As he dialed, he felt confident that the doctor would give Marilyn a clean report. He was even imagining himself giving Marilyn the reassuring news when Dr. Roberts came on the line.

"Dave, the barium enema and gallbladder X-rays are all fine," said the radiologist. He hesitated, then proceeded in an unmistakably solemn tone. "The upper G.I. reveals a four-by-eight centimeter mass on the fundus of the stomach. It looks benign, but I can't be sure. I advise you to get your wife to a gastroenterologist soon."

"You found a tumor?" David replied numbly. He paused a moment before adding, "I—I'll come by and pick up the X-rays and hand-deliver them myself."

In a daze David hung up the phone and stumbled into the darkened staff lounge behind his office. He fell on his chest and wept bitterly. "Dear God, what now!" he cried. "*Why* now?" The torment welled up inside him. He wanted to pound his fists on the floor. "Oh, God, not Marilyn," he pleaded. "My body, my own body has been broken, and I have my limitations, but please not Marilyn!" He stared up into the darkness, his face wet with tears. "God, why don't you just take me? I can't live on the brink of family and personal catastrophe forever. I just can't continue on the edge of death!"

As David poured out his need, his devastation, his

mother's words unexpectedly flashed in his mind. "Son, God has chosen you for a special work." When had Margarita spoken those words? Then he remembered. It was during his spiritual crisis just before graduating from medical school. In desperation he had telephoned his mother from a public phone booth. She had said, "David, consider yourself an important part of God's history for the universe. God loves you. We love you. Do you love him?"

David sat up, removed his metal-rimmed glasses, and wiped his eyes. "Yes, God, I love you," he murmured. "But I don't understand. Would you bring us to this place merely to drop us, to abandon us?"

The answer came to David as if God were actually speaking the words: "My grace is sufficient for thee; for my strength is made perfect in weakness."

David methodically rubbed his hand over his face and jaw. "Well, if it is sufficient, dear God, I'm in a crisis of trust right now. I need to know just now that you love us, that you care for us, that you will get us through this episode. I need to know that you are here, in Pasadena, at 3:45 in the afternoon, imbuing me with your grace." He sighed deeply, almost a shudder, and added, "And, Father, please, I need strength to break the news to Marilyn."

He stood up then, the tears spent. He felt cleansed somehow; the oppressiveness was lifting. He sensed God's peace, an inexplicable washing of the wound that moments ago had seemed beyond healing. The anguish had dissipated. That feeling that he was living on the edge of catastrophe was gone. Instead, he felt suddenly as if he were standing on the edge of something beautiful, on the margin of a personal miracle, the perimeter of a family triumph.

"Father, I know now that you won't take me at this particular time," he said earnestly. "I believe you want me to be part of that special blessing you have planned for our family. Help us now to reactivate our faith . . . a faith that has already been tried in the fires of suffering. Help us to reignite our trust . . . to be still and know that you are God."

David washed his face, cleaned his glasses and straightened his tie, then returned to his patients. When he had seen the last one, he telephoned a specialist and made an appointment for Marilyn at nine-thirty the next morning.

The drive home was burdensome as David rehearsed in his mind what he would tell Marilyn. His dear Marilyn! The center of beauty in their home, the one who brought stability to their lives in spite of David's illness. How he treasured her warmth, her steady, loving care, her selfless devotion to him and the boys. How could he possibly tell her of the tumor?

On his arrival home, David and Marilyn greeted each other as usual with a smile and a kiss. Then she asked, "Have you heard from the radiologist?"

David was momentarily silent. Then, walking with her into the living room, he said, "Yes, sweetheart."

"Well, what did he say?" she asked, sitting down.

He joined her, slipping his arm around her shoulder. "All is well, except for a possible tumor," he said, trying to sound casual. "It's resting on top of the stomach. It appears benign."

Marilyn looked searchingly at him. "Oh, David . . . a tumor?"

The import of his words struck him afresh. He broke down. Marilyn, too, began to cry. They held each other reassuringly.

Suddenly Michael and Mark, in striped polo shirts and jeans, bounded into the room and stopped abruptly. "Why are you two crying?" Michael asked innocently, pushing his sea captain's hat back on his straight dark brown hair.

David and Marilyn opened their arms tenderly to include their sons in the family circle of grief.

On Thursday morning, Margarita Hernandez flew down from San Jose to be with David and Marilyn. David picked her up at eight A.M. Then he took Marilyn in for another consultation and had her X-rays reviewed by another radiologist, who made the same diagnosis as Dr. Roberts.

That evening David telephoned Pastor Lee and said, "Tomorrow morning Marilyn will enter the hospital and have a gastroscopy to inspect the interior of the stomach. We don't know what they'll find."

"Well, Dave, all of us in the Early Christians Prayer Group will be praying for her at that time," Pastor Lee assured him.

On Friday morning David and Marilyn left for the hospital at seven A.M. In their haste they forgot to leave the car keys to the Volkswagen with Margarita so that she could drive the boys to school at eight-thirty. She telephoned Marilyn's parents, who promptly picked up the boys and delivered them to the San Gabriel Christian Elementary School.

At the hospital, before the procedure, David gently reassured Marilyn that everything would be all right, that God was with them. Marilyn smiled faintly. "I know. It's just that things seem to be happening so rapidly in our lives. One event merges with the next before we can even catch up."

Nevertheless, Marilyn remained so calm and tolerated the gastroscopy so well that she and David knew the Lord was in control. But the physician reported that no lesion was visible and a biopsy was impossible. He suggested, "Why don't you wait two weeks and repeat the upper G.I. X-ray with special air contrast techniques?"

Reluctantly David and Marilyn agreed. They left the hospital at nine-fifteen and began the drive to David's office. On the way he glanced at her and said, "You know, hon, I don't feel like waiting two weeks. You haven't had breakfast yet, so why don't we repeat the X-ray this morning—if I can get the radiologist at Huntington Memorial to do it."

Marilyn shrugged and said, "Whatever you think."

When David telephoned the radiologist, the doctor replied, "Dave, we're up to our necks with work, but if you get your wife right over, we'll process her."

That afternoon the radiologists at Huntington Memorial examined Marilyn's X-rays and concluded that she had a large stomach tumor, probably benign. David called Dr. Baldridge, Vic Herlacher's associate, with a specialty in gastroenterology at Huntington Memorial. He studied the films and advised a surgery consultation, which he scheduled for Monday.

The weekend proved to be a quixotic misadventure for the entire Hernandez family. On Friday evening, after showering in the guest bathroom, Margarita discovered that she couldn't turn off the shower valve. Frantically she threw on her bathrobe and summoned David, who managed after much effort to turn off the hot water; but the cold water remained inexorably stuck. Finally, in desperation, he stalked to the basement and turned off the master valve. It solved the problem of the excess water; but now there was no water at all.

David turned the valve on briefly Saturday morning to refill the toilet tanks and telephoned the plumber; then he drove his mother to the airport for her return to San Jose. Later, another minor crisis erupted when the washing machine malfunctioned, forcing Marilyn to take all the laundry to a laundromat. To make matters worse, when she transferred the wet clothes to a plastic bag, the bottom gave out, spilling the clean garments all over the grimy linoleum floor.

The one bright spot on Saturday occurred when Pastor Lee dropped by to visit and pray with the family. As usual, everyone was blessed by the pastor's loving spirit and warm concern.

Sunday morning arrived with rain and gloom. Because it was Mother's Day, Dee served David and Marilyn breakfast in bed. Then after church David took the family to a Chinese restaurant for lunch. The food was delightful; but as the family walked toward the parking lot, David asked Marilyn, "Where are my keys, Babe?"

"Don't you remember?" she said tolerantly. "They're so bulky that I offered to carry them for you in my purse."

He gave her a scrutinizing glance. "Then where's your purse?"

Marilyn looked down in dismay. "My purse—it's gone!"

"Where did you see it last?" cried Dee.

Marilyn groaned. "In the car."

Sure enough, the keys were locked in the automobile. Marilyn shivered in the chill wind as David gazed woefully at the dark clouds gathering overhead.

"I'll walk home and get the other set of keys," offered Dee. The boys applauded.

"I'll go with you, Auntie Dee!" exclaimed Mark.

"Me too. Me too!" shouted Michael.

David smiled ironically. "You might know. Walking ten blocks home sounds like fun to them. But go on, if you wish."

So the hearty threesome started off toward home while David and Marilyn stood shivering together in the cold.

The family braved the elements again to attend the evening service at church, where Ann Kiemel would be speaking. Before the service, David and Marilyn met with their close friends Jim Dobson and Vic Herlacher for prayer. They felt themselves strengthened immeasurably by their friends' love and support.

On Monday morning Marilyn underwent a surgery consultation and additional tests, including an intravenous pyelogram and several blood tests. Surgery was scheduled for ten A.M. on Tuesday.

David arrived at the hospital early the next morning to spend some time with Marilyn. He was encouraged to see her smiling.

"How's it going, sweetheart?" he asked, kissing her.

"I'm okay," she said softly. "I really am. God has given me such a peace about everything."

"I'm so glad," he said.

"David, you know what has really helped me? The miracle God worked in my mother's life last year."

"You mean when she had her massive heart attack?"

"Yes," said Marilyn. "Remember? I telephoned her that morning and she was having pains. I drove over immediately and took her to the hospital. The doctor said if I hadn't gotten her there so quickly, she would have died."

David nodded. "God was certainly watching over her. He allowed you to call her and drive over at just the right moment."

"And now he's taking care of *me* too," Marilyn murmured. "I know he is, David."

At nine-thirty Marilyn was wheeled into the operating room. David was in attendance to observe the procedure. A half hour into surgery, Dr. Johnston, the surgeon, gave David a sober, concerned glance. David could see why. There before them were two contiguous tumors measuring about four-by-ten-by-six centimeters. The masses sat on top of the stomach and involved the left segment of the liver. Dr. Johnston explored the stomach thoroughly, and found the situation to be completely negative.

David's thoughts raced ahead of the surgeon. *Is this a primary lesion of the liver? It looks ominous and malignant. If it's secondary, where is the primary lesion?* As he considered the possibilities, David's confidence began to falter.

Dr. Johnston remained silently engrossed in his exploration of the questionable area. He felt carefully, skillfully for lymph nodes, then checked the bowel and pelvis for other lesions. "All appears clear," he announced, "but we'll attempt removal of the most accessible mass and do a rapid frozen section for the pathologist. We'll wait for his verdict, then decide how much more surgery will be required and how radical our procedure must be."

The surgeon resected the first tumor and handed David the specimen. David rushed it upstairs to the pathologist. As Dr. Arthur Koehler, a colleague and friend from Loma Linda University, studied the specimen, David was struck with the unnerving realization that within a few minutes he would be receiving news of profound import. The essence of life and death swung in the balance. The wonderful years of his marriage with Marilyn flashed in his mind's eye. He was accosted by the devastating vision of his sons Mark and Michael threatened again by the loss of a parent. The minutes slogged by, unbearably slow. David reflected on the reality of life and of death, and thanked God again for the reality of life after death.

As Art placed a slide under the microscope, David whispered a brief prayer. Moments later, Art signaled for David to come view the slide. "What do you think, Dave?" he questioned. He was smiling.

"It looks benign," said David, his voice weak with relief.

"I agree," said Art. "Let's go tell O.R."

Following the pathologist's report, Dr. Johnston proceeded with the operation, resecting about ten to fifteen percent of the left segment of the liver. As David watched, he recognized that Marilyn wasn't out of danger yet. He knew by personal experience that liver surgery was often precarious. The liver was a vital organ and surgery could be complicated by infection, hemorrhage, bile leakage, or peritonitis. And Marilyn's diabetes would likely make recovery even more difficult.

As David suspected, Marilyn's recovery was onerous and hard-won. But with slow, persistent effort and care, she regained her strength. During those days of inching back to normalcy, David and Marilyn claimed Isaiah 43:2 as God's special promise to them: "When thou passest through the waters, I will be with thee; and through the rivers, they shall not overflow thee: when thou walkest through the fire, thou shalt not be burned; neither shall the flame kindle upon thee."

Both David and Marilyn had come through the perilous waters of physical vulnerability and through the fires of personal testing; they had confronted the malignant specter of death and survived. Their weaknesses, their limitations, their humanity—exposed and fallible—had been bathed miraculously in God's boundless grace. Together they praised God.

TWENTY-SEVEN

In the fall of 1978, David was presented with a unique and challenging opportunity to appear on Dr. Jim Dobson's new television series being videotaped in Chicago. The program "Focus on the Family," named after Jim's Arcadia-based organization dedicated to the preservation of the home, was being prepared for national syndication.

David and Marilyn discussed the extraordinary prospect at some length one evening while she prepared dinner. Helping himself to a wedge of avocado from the salad Marilyn was tossing, David said, "It looks like Jim and the Domain Advertising Agency will be paying our way to Chicago to tape three shows."

"Our way?" echoed Marilyn. "You mean they want me to go too?"

"Sure, hon. I wouldn't go without you."

Marilyn carried the salad bowl to the dining room table. "I'm sorry, David, but no one's going to get me on TV."

He was right behind her. "You don't have to be, sweetheart. You can sit in the audience and watch."

She eyed him suspiciously. "You're sure?"

"Positive."

"Then I'd love to go," she beamed. She returned to the kitchen for a platter of roast beef and vegetables. Coming back, she said, "Is Shirley [Jim's wife] going too?"

David smiled. "Of course. Where would we men be without our wives?"

"Not in Chicago," said Marilyn teasingly. She brightened at another thought. "Shirley and I can go shopping!"

David shook his head in mock dismay. "What would you girls do if you couldn't shop?"

"Don't be smart," she countered. "You guys will be too busy to notice us anyway." She nudged him playfully as she returned to the kitchen for the biscuits.

At dinner they were still talking about the upcoming television show. The boys were fascinated at the prospect of Daddy being on TV.

"Won't you be scared?" Mark asked soberly.

"Will you be famous, Daddy?" questioned Michael, his light green eyes dancing. "As famous as . . . as Tarzan and the Super Seven?"

David looked bewildered. "Tarzan and who?"

"The Super Seven," explained Mark. "But that's dumb. They're cartoons!"

"They're not dumb!" insisted Michael, making a face.

"Maybe we'd better continue this discussion after dinner," suggested David, giving the boys a glance that said, *behave!*

Later, after the boys were in bed, David and Marilyn sat together, relaxing before the fireplace. "Just what does Jim want you to do on these programs?" Marilyn asked.

"He gave me three topics," said David, "one for each show."

Marilyn gazed questioningly at him. "On—?"

"First, on women's medical problems—menopause, post-partum depression, that sort of thing. The second has to do with marital problems and sexuality. And the third show will be my testimony."

"How do you really feel about doing the programs?"

David looked thoughtful. "You know I'm not afraid of public speaking. I've lectured at service clubs, youth clinics, and health classes—"

"Not to mention family planning councils, hospital committee meetings, and church programs," added Marilyn.

David's brow furrowed. He adjusted his glasses, more out

of habit than need. "But a program like 'Focus on the Family' requires humor, perfect timing, and the ability to entertain while conveying a message. And you can't preach. The show is geared to a secular audience, so religious jargon is out. Sponsors won't touch it if it even smells evangelical."

"It sounds like it's going to be hard," sighed Marilyn.

"There's more," he said. "Jim says they do the program in seven and nine-minute segments. So how, in a few short minutes, are you going to entertain and get God's message across on touchy subjects?"

"I can't begin to imagine—"

"There's still more. We'll have a live audience, and there will be a question and answer period. I'll have no way of knowing what questions they'll ask and no way to prepare my answers."

Marilyn eased comfortably into David's arms. "Honey, do you think you should tell Jim you can't do it?"

"Oh, I'll do it, Babe. It's just a tremendous burden on me, knowing that they have so much money invested in this thing. I wouldn't want to do anything to make it all go down the drain."

"You won't," she assured him. "The Lord will make it go just right."

On October 26, 1978, David and Marilyn flew to Chicago for the tapings. Early the next morning, Marilyn and Shirley, Jim's wife, left for a day of shopping at Marshall Fields. Actually, David and Jim, anxious for time alone to plan their strategy for the evening's programs, sent the girls promptly on their way.

"We'll be taping three shows, one after another," said Jim, "and we have only today to get it together."

For two hours they talked with sober concentration. Finally Jim said, "I think we've done enough homework, Dave. What do you think?"

David nodded in relief. "It sounds good, Jim. I'm going to my room to pray and think for a while." He didn't dare add that an irrational sense of panic had taken root inside him. Somehow, before showtime, he had to dispel it.

An hour later, the two men caught a taxi to the television studio. David remained silent all the way, vainly trying to subdue his mushrooming terror. He knew his nervousness was obvious; usually he and Jim talked together constantly. To David's consternation, the taxi driver, a young Korean, traveled at a leisurely pace, as if he had all day and didn't mind spending it with his two passengers. In fact, Jim and the man had become engrossed in conversation; they seemed perfectly delighted with each other's company.

David groaned inwardly. He had hoped to arrive at the studio in time to relax a little, become acquainted with the cameras and the set, and grab a bite to eat. He and Jim had worked so diligently, they had taken no time for lunch. Now David's blood sugar was precariously low.

At last, after a seemingly endless drive, the taxi pulled up in front of the studio. As David and Jim left the cab, Jim handed the driver the fare with a fifteen percent tip. The man was all grin until his eyes scanned the amount in his hand. His face fell. He glared accusingly at Jim and said, "Aw, I should have known you were going to give me a small tip."

Jim stared back dumbfounded. "I've never had anyone complain about a fifteen percent tip," he said.

"Yeah? Well, you talk buddy-buddy," retorted the man, "until it comes to your wallet!"

Jim was shocked by the driver's irritated reaction. He pivoted and strode briskly after David.

As soon as the two entered the studio, they were greeted by Gil Moegerle, co-host and producer of the program, and Pat McMillan, the program consultant and co-producer. (Pat is also the award-winning producer of the popular "Phil Donahue Show.") Minutes later, they were ushered to a set and asked to sit on stools while the cameramen adjusted their cameras. After a half hour of waiting, Jim grew impatient. "What's taking so long?" he asked.

"We have only three cameras. We need four," replied one cameraman. "When we zoom in on one of you, we hide the other."

(David learned afterward that his own awkward silence backstage had caused everyone to assume that he was something of a noncommunicative dud. Figuring he would sit in his place and not move a muscle, they were feverishly trying to set the camera angles close to capture him at his best.)

Finally David leaned over and whispered urgently, "Jim, we've got to get out of here."

Jim nodded and stood up, lifting his hands for attention. "Folks, this is only creating more tension," he said. "Can you guys get a substitute for Dr. Hernandez and myself? Then you can work on your cameras all you please."

"OK, bring in two other men," Gil called wearily.

In relief David and Jim left the set and walked to the back of the studio. They went over their material again, briefly, then had a light dinner. David couldn't eat much. His nerves were playing havoc with his stomach.

Twenty minutes before the first taping, they went backstage to wait. David felt weak. His mind was closing; he couldn't think straight. He realized in dismay that he was suffering a mental block; he couldn't even recall the topics to be discussed!

"I don't know how we're going to get this thing rolling," he said miserably. What he really wanted to say was, *Put me on a stretcher and carry me out of this place!*

Jim gave him a penetrating glance. "Dave, let's pray about this." Bowing his head, Jim said, "Lord, you know that we aren't here for our own glory. We're not here to make money. We're here because we think we have a message that has come from you. There's no way in the world that we can in our own strength do this thing and do it right. We just beg you to take over."

By the time Jim said, "Amen," David was beginning to feel a sense of well-being. They exchanged a comradely grin, then Jim walked out on stage before the blinding spotlights. While the cameras rolled, Gil, the co-host and announcer, introduced Jim. They shook hands; then Jim introduced David. David felt a bit stiff, but he hoped that things were proceeding smoothly enough. Then, without warning, one of the cameras malfunctioned.

"We've got to take it again," Pat, the co-producer, interrupted.

Quelling their frustration, David and Jim exited. When Gil repeated the introduction, they made their entrance again. At least David was more relaxed this time. But once more the camera refused to operate.

"One more time," called Pat, her voice tinged with frustration.

"Pat, you're just going to have to edit it," said Jim firmly. "We're a half hour behind and we have three shows to do."

"Jim, we can't do it," said Pat. "We can't edit it; we don't have anything recorded yet."

"Why not?" asked Jim impatiently.

"The third camera has blown. We need a new one."

"It'll take at least thirty minutes to bring in another camera," Jim said in exasperation. "We can't hold the audience for that long."

"That's right," came the reply.

Jim heaved a sigh, then waved his hand toward the audience in a gesture of dismissal. "Maybe you'd like to get a cup of coffee or something. We'll try again shortly."

By the time the new camera was adjusted and warmed up, Jim was distressed. The taping had been delayed nearly an hour; now they had only two hours to complete three shows, and they were starting with a tired audience.

Surprisingly, David was feeling much better now. The delays that had annoyed Jim had provided David with much needed "dry runs" to help dispel his fears.

But the irritations weren't over yet. According to plan, as the cameras rolled David and Jim walked on stage and talked together. Then they were allotted one minute to take their chairs and put on their microphones before the cameras swung back their way. Unfortunately, when they reached their seats they found their microphones badly tangled. The camera focused on them just as they fumbled awkwardly with the snarled cords. What else could they do but look up and grin sheepishly into that relentless, all-revealing eye?

After that, things proceeded smoothly. David, his fears gone, felt himself in perfect contact with the audience. He gestured freely, speaking with relaxed authority. Then, unexpectedly, a cameraman signaled a break and announced, "Dr. Hernandez, we just can't keep up with you. We've got to reset the cameras."

They broke for a couple of minutes, repositioned the cameras, then resumed the show. When they completed the first program, they went on immediately to the second. David was bombarded with a variety of questions from the studio audience. Couples asked confidential questions about their sex life, love-making techniques, and problems relating to physical compatibility. After one intimate question, David glanced hopefully at Jim to see if he would like to attempt an answer, but with a nod Jim gave it back to him. Then the producer signaled that he had three minutes remaining.

Think fast, David told himself. *This night is costing thousands of dollars to tape and hundreds of dollars an hour to edit. Don't blow it now!* He began to speak, addressing the needs of this particular couple, and the words flowed effortlessly. Suddenly Gil signaled fifteen seconds to close. David made a concluding remark. Then came the wrap-up signal. *Five seconds.* David finished his reply just as he received the signal to cut.

They finished the second show at 9:45 P.M. Jim turned to Pat McMillan and said, "We're supposed to be out of here by ten. I guess we'll have to forego the last program."

"No, go ahead," said Pat. "Get it down now."

Jim nodded and turned confidentially to David. "The big question concerns this last episode."

"Why?" asked David. "You'll be interviewing me, won't you? I'll just be giving my testimony."

"It's not called a testimony," said Jim quickly. "That would not fit the theme of the program, which is meaningful family life. We want to hear how your family coped with life's stresses."

On that note the third program began. David talked of his Mexican heritage, about his grandfathers Jesus and Jose Maria and their bitter struggles to survive against overwhelming odds; about his parents Jose and Margarita, their poverty and relentless efforts to improve life for themselves and their children. As he spoke, David sensed that he had the audience with him, listening to every word.

But at the half-way mark, during the one-minute break,

Pat approached Gil Moegerle and whispered, "This can't go on."

Gil stared at her in surprise. "What do you mean?"

"I mean," said Pat, "it's a nice, folksy little story, but the TV audience won't go for it. It won't go over on national television."

"What do you want me to do then?" asked Gil.

"Go over and tell Jim we might as well quit taping."

Gil nodded reluctantly and relayed the message to Jim Dobson, who strongly disagreed with Pat's assessment. Just then, Gil received the signal, *Five seconds.* The lights blared suddenly and the cameras went on and focused again on Gil, then on Jim and David.

Jim turned to David and said, "Dave, would you tell us something about your recent illness and the stresses your family encountered?"

David launched into a brief recounting of the events surrounding his rare ailment and the effect it had had on his family and himself. "In the midst of this experience," he added, "I wrestled with the Lord and, like Jacob of old, I said to him, 'I will not let you go until you bless me.' I didn't know whether the blessing would be physical healing or spiritual renewal or just the peace that passes all understanding. I have God's peace, and I trust him for tomorrow." He hesitated, trying to see out into the audience, but the lights were too blinding.

"I know that miracles are a means to God's ends," he continued, his voice wavering slightly, "but God's ends have to do with making men, not making magic. There is as much miracle in roses, in breathing and babies as there is in falling manna, or the Red Sea split open, or a lame man healed by the pool of Bethesda."

David took a breath and looked around earnestly. "In the time remaining to me—be it months or years or decades—I will enjoy life to the fullest and be grateful. I will appreciate the simple things around me—the trees and greenery, the sunshine and the rain, the magic of growing things."

A wave of emotion caught David unawares and he looked over at Jim, hoping he would say something while David composed himself. It startled him to see that Jim, a strapping, self-contained man, was fighting back tears, too choked up to speak.

So David continued. "When I was growing up, my father taught me an enduring sense of self-reliance. But more important than that, my Heavenly Father has taught me an enduring sense of *God-reliance*."

At that moment the co-producer signaled the three-minute wrap-up. David looked at Gil, who took over and turned the program back to Jim. Jim spoke over rising emotion. A minute passed. He could no longer continue. He turned back to David and said, "Do you have anything else to say?"

The one-minute signal.

David blinked back tears and said, "Survival has been an important word to my family. Survival in this life . . . survival of the family unit . . . survival after death. My family—my wife, my two sons, my parents—they have kept me going in the face of despair. I love them; I praise God for them. I depend on them more than I can say. They have taught me how to survive. But I have learned that ultimately the only means of genuine survival any of us has is Jesus Christ. That's why I can say with the Apostle Paul, 'To me to live is Christ, and to die is gain.' "

The five-second wrap-up. . . . Cut!

The hot, glaring lights dimmed; the cameras moved back into the shadows; the audience, almost *en masse*, surrounded the set. People were weeping; many extended their hands to David in compassion and friendship. All appeared visibly moved.

Meanwhile, the co-producer approached Gil and asked urgently, "Did you tell him?"

"Pat, Jim felt we should continue."

"Oh, no, that's not what I meant," she said with unabashed enthusiasm. "I was hoping that you hadn't gotten to him. I think that was one of the best programs I've ever seen!"

David greeted dozens of people, exchanging warm words of appreciation and encouragement. But within minutes his eyes searched beyond the crowd—for Marilyn. She was standing off to one side, smiling, her eyes glistening. He made his way through the throng and took her in his arms. *God is good*, he thought, marveling. The rest of the world seemed to recede obligingly—the lights, the noises, the rustling, passing, effusive humanity. For one long moment he held her wordlessly, with profound love and gratitude, as if he would never let her go.

EPILOGUE

As I "rest" anxiously in the doctor's "sleeping room," I await word on the outcome of my father's surgery. My patient is in labor, but my mind is on my dad. Memories of his life and example flow unbidden through my mind. A man of energy and strength, afraid of nothing, not known to moan or complain, he is now recovering from a heart attack, dependent on a pacemaker for his survival.

My admiration for this man can be matched only by my love for him. I whisper a little prayer and commit him again to our loving heavenly Father. I feel peace.

I thank God I am part of a family that faithfully surrounds its members with incredible support and prayer. My family has often come to my rescue. My thoughts remind me of a story I once heard.

A man dreamed he was walking along a beach with the Lord as scenes from his life flashed across the sky. When the final scene finished, he looked back and noticed that at some points in his life there was only one set of footprints in the sand, and this was consistently during the lowest, saddest times in his life. "Lord, you promised to always be with me. Why did you desert me when I needed you most?" "My child, I love you and will never abandon you. During your hardest moments I carried you."

God has often carried members of my family through times of hardship and failure. He broke into our lives with his power and love. That is our story.